1672

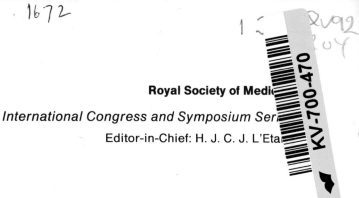

Royal Society of Medic

International Congress and Symposium Ser

Editor-in-Chief: H. J. C. J. L'Eta

Number 64

Advances in morphine therapy

The 1983 international symposium on pain control

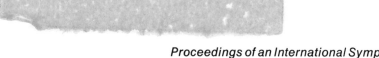

*Proceedings of an International Symposium
sponsored by Napp Laboratories, held
in Geneva, 14–16 October 1983*

Royal Society of Medicine

International Congress and Symposium Series

Number 64

Advances in morphine therapy

The 1983 international symposium on pain control

Edited by

E. Wilkes
J. Levy

1984

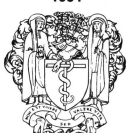

Published by

The Royal Society of Medicine
1 Wimpole Street, London

ROYAL SOCIETY OF MEDICINE

1 Wimpole Street, London W1M 8AE

Distributed by

OXFORD UNIVERSITY PRESS
Walton Street, Oxford OX2 6DP

London New York Toronto
Delhi Bombay Calcutta Madras Karachi
Kuala Lumpur Singapore Hong Kong Tokyo
Nairobi Dar es Salaam Cape Town
Melbourne Auckland

and associated companies in
Beirut Berlin Ibadan Mexico City Nicosia

Oxford is a trade mark of Oxford University Press

Copyright © 1984 by

ROYAL SOCIETY OF MEDICINE

British Library Cataloguing in Publication Data

Advances in morphine therapy.—(International
congress and symposium series/Royal Society
of Medicine; no. 64)
1. Morphine   2. Analgesia
I. Wilkes, Eric   II. Series
616′.0472   RM666.M8
ISBN 0–19–922007–7

Library of Congress Cataloging in Publication Data

International Symposium on Pain Control (1983: Geneva, Switzerland)
Advances in morphine therapy.
(International congress and symposium series; no. 64)
'Proceedings of an international symposium sponsored by Napp Laboratories, in Geneva':
1. Pain—Chemotherapy—Congresses.   2. Morphine—Therapeutic use—Congresses.   3. Pain, Postoperative—Chemotherapy—Congresses.   4. Terminal care—Congresses.
I. Wilkes, Eric, 1920-   .   II. Napp Laboratories.   III. Title.   IV. Series. [DNLM: 1. Morphinans—pharmacodynamics—congresses.   2. Anesthesiology—congresses.
W3 IN207 no. 65/QV 92 B944 1982]
RB127.I583 1983   616′.0472   84–7198
ISBN 0–19–922007–7

Printed in Great Britain at the University Press, Oxford

Contributors

Professor J. Ammon
    Med. Einrichtungen der RWTH Aachen, Universitatsklinikum Radiologie, D 5100 Aachen

Dr R. Assaf
    Consultant Anaesthetist, St. Vincent's Hospital, Elm Park, Dublin 4

Dr I. M. C. Clarke
    Director, North West Pain Centre, Hope Hospital, Eccles Old Road, Salford, Lancs

Professor M. Chayen
    Khilat Padua 12, Tel Aviv, Israel

Dr R. J. Dickson
    Consultant Radiotherapist, Mount Vernon Hospital, Sir Michael Sobell House, Northwood, Middlesex

Professor A. Doenicke
    Chirug. Univ. Klinik u. Poliklinik, Munchen-Innenstadt, Pettenkoferstrasse 8a, D 800, Munchen 2

Professor H. U. Gerbershagen
    Schmerz-Zentrum Mainz, 65 Mainz

Dr N. H. Gordon
    Consultant Anaesthetist, Western General Hospital, Crewe Road, Edinburgh

Dr E. G. Hadaway
    Consultant Anaesthetist, Kettering General Hospital, Rothwell Road, Kettering, Northants

Dr G. Hanks
    Consultant Physician, Royal Marsden Hospital, Fulham Road, London

Professor H. Henriksen
    Department of Anaesthesia, Finsen Institute, Copenhagen, Denmark

Dr T. Hunt
    Senior Clinical Medical Officer, Sir Arthur Rank House, Brookfields Hospital, Mill Road, Cambridge

Mr P. Jarrett
    Consultant Surgeon, Kingston Hospital, Galsworthy Road, Kingston upon Thames, Surrey

Professor I. Jurna
    Inst. fur Pharmakologie u. Toxikologie, der Universität des Saarlandes, D 6650 Homburg/Saar

Dr B. Kay
Senior Lecturer in Anaesthetics, Withington Hospital, West Didsbury, Manchester

Dr A. Kimberley
Senior Registrar in Anaesthetics, Westminster Hospital, Dean Ryle Street, London

Dr B. Kossman
Sentrum fur Anasthesiologie, Universitatskliniken Ulm, Prillwitzstrasse 43, Ulm, Germany

Dr R. Lamerton
16 Whitehall Park, London, N16

Dr J. Levy
Napp Laboratories Limited, Cambridge Science Park, Milton Road, Cambridge

Dr H. McQuay
Nuffield Departments of Anaesthetics and Clinical Biochemistry, The Radcliffe Infirmary, Oxford

Dr G. Park
Consultant Anaesthetist, Addenbrooke's Hospital, Hills Road, Cambridge

Dr F. Randell
Macmillan Continuing Care Unit, Christchurch Hospital, Christchurch, Dorset

Dr C. B. Regnard
Sir Michael Sobell House, The Churchill Hospital, Headington, Oxford

Dr H. Slowey
Lecturer in Anaesthesia, University Hospital of Wales, Heath Park, Cardiff, CF4 4XY

Professor G. Smith
Professor of Anaesthesia, University of Leicester, Leicester

Professor V. Ventafridda
Scientific Director, Fondazione Floriani, Viccolo Fiore 2, I 20121 Milano

Dr T. D. Walsh
Fellow in Clinical Pharmacology, St. Christopher's Hospice, 51–53 Lawrie Park Road, Sydenham, London

Miss D. Watson
Consultant Surgeon, East Birmingham Hospital, Bordesley Green, Birmingham, B9 5ST

Contents

Session 1: Perioperative pain control

Chairmen

M. BAUM

M. D. VICKERS

The pharmacology of pain control
Multi-level action of analgesic agents

I. JURNA

Institut für Pharmakologie und Toxikologie der Universität des Saarlandes,
Homburg/Saar,
Federal Republic of Germany

Not very long ago most people thought that pain processing was exclusively a matter of the brain. In accordance with this view, analgesic agents were assumed to depress pain sensation as well as any kind of response evoked by painful stimuli by an action on the brain. However, in the course of the last 10 years we have learned that this is not true. Drugs used in the management of pain, i.e. analgesic agents proper, central muscle relaxants, neuroleptic and antidepressant agents may cause relief from pain by acting at different levels of that part of the nervous system which is known as the nociceptive system.

Tissue damage by injury or inflammatory processes induces the formation and release of bradykinin, histamine 5-hydroxytryptamine, and prostaglandin E_2 (Fig. 1). These analgesic substances activate nociceptors (Handwerker 1980) which are the peripheral terminals of primary nociceptive afferents. Activation of nociceptors generates impulses which are conducted by primary nociceptive afferents consisting of myelinated $A\delta$ fibres and unmyelinated C fibres. Primary nociceptive afferents mostly terminate in the substantia gelatinosa of the dorsal horn, where they make synaptic contact with neurones participating in either motor or sensory responses of the spinal nociceptive system.

Motor responses or nociceptive reflexes are based upon flexor reflex activity elicited by ipsilateral noxious stimulation, and on concomitant crossed extensor reflexes supporting flexor reflexes. These responses manifest themselves as withdrawal reflexes or local tonic muscle contractions.

The sensory response consists in activity set up in ascending axons of the classical pain pathway in the spinal cord, the spinothalamic tract (Fig. 1). This leads to changes in parameters of the autonomic nervous system (e.g. heart rate, blood pressure, respiration, perspiration, etc.), wakefulness, emotional and affective behaviour, and, above all, the sensation of pain and its transfer from a physiological phenomenon into subjective experience which is probably achieved by projections to the frontal lobe.

Prostaglandin E_2 does not activate nociceptors but is prerequisite to stimulation of nociceptors (Ferreira *et al.* 1974; Moncada *et al.* 1975). In the absence of

Advances in Morphine Therapy. The 1983 International Symposium on Pain Control, edited by E. Wilkes, 1984: Royal Society of Medicine International Congress and Symposium Series No. 64, published by the Royal Society of Medicine.

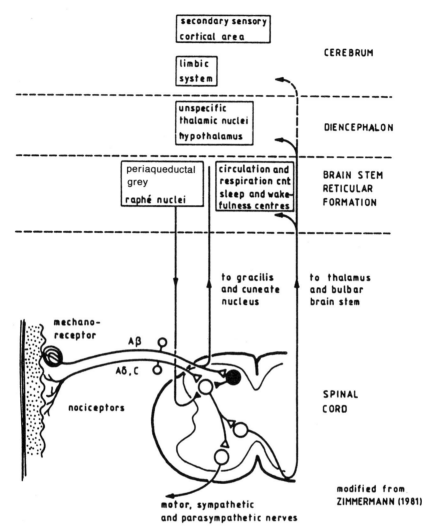

Fig. 1. Schematic diagram of the spinal nociceptive system. Nociceptors are peripheral endings of nociceptive afferents (Aδ and C fibres). These afferents terminate mostly in the substantia gelatinosa of the spinal cord, where they make synaptic contact with neurones either forming part of motor reflex paths (flexor reflex path; crossed extensor reflex path, not shown) and autonomic reflex paths, or sending their axons in the spinothalamic tract to the brain. Impulse transmission from nociceptive afferents is inhibited from the brainstem by descending path (black terminal) and an endorphinergic neurone (black soma and terminal). Hypothetically, the endorphinergic neurone is activated by a non-nociceptive afferent (Aβ fibre).

prostaglandin E_2, the sensitivity of nociceptors to bradykinin, histamine or 5-hydroxytryptamine is much reduced. The level of prostaglandin E_2 in injured or inflamed tissue is lowered by corticosteroids, non-steroidal anti-inflammatory drugs of the acetylsalicylic acid (or aspirin) type (Flower 1974).

Thus, corticosteroids and non-steroidal anti-inflammatory drugs will reduce the impulse input to the central nervous system (Handwerker 1976) and, consequently, abolish the sensation of pain. Because of this mode of action, non-steroidal anti-inflammatory drugs are often termed 'peripherally acting analgesic agents', as opposed to 'centrally acting analgesic agents' of the morphine type. Although corticosteroids also reduce the content of prostaglandin E_2, they fail to produce analgesia unless the cause of pain is tissue damage or inflammation. Nobody will use them instead of acetylsalicylic acid to cure a headache caused by a hangover. Very likely, salicylic acid, pyrazol, and aniline derivatives such as aspirin, metamizol or paracetamol diminish pain sensation also by a central site of action.

By reducing the nociceptive impulse input, corticosteroids and non-steroidal anti-inflammatory drugs depress nociceptive reflex activity and the 'wind-up' due to painful tonic muscle stretch and pull at tendons and ligaments in myalgia and ischialgia.

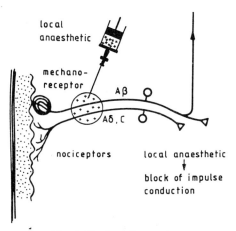

Fig. 2. Nociceptive system.

Blocking impulse conduction in primary nociceptive afferents by applying local anaesthetics is a very simple and effective means to switch-off pain sensation (Fig. 2). It has the disadvantage of blocking all sensory afferents. The discovery of opiate receptors on primary nociceptive afferents (Fields *et al.* 1980) as well as the observation that morphine depresses impulse conduction in these nerve fibres (Jurna and Grossmann 1977) suggest that a reduced nociceptive impulse input may contribute to the beneficial effect of locally (intrathecally) or systemically administered morphine.

The substantia gelatinosa of the spinal cord dorsal horn, where impulses are transmitted from the terminals of primary nociceptive afferents to secondary neurones of the nociceptive system, is rich in opiate receptors and their endogenous ligandes metenkephalin and dynorphin (Atweh and Kuhar 1983; Cuello 1983). When these peptides are released from endorphinergic neurones, impulse transmission from primary nociceptive afferents is blocked (Duggan *et al.* 1977). This also happens when the opiate receptors in this region are occupied when morphine is administered systemically (Duggan *et al.* 1977b; Jurna and Heinz 1979) or into the cerebrospinal fluid (Doi and Jurna 1982). The latter mode of application, which is used clinically to produce spinal analgesia, selectively blocks pain sensation and nociceptive reflex activity without affecting other sensations and voluntary movement.

Before reaching their destination in unspecific thalamic nuclei, the ascending axons of the spinothalamic tract send collaterals into the reticular formation of the brainstem. By means of these collaterals, changes in autonomic nervous function and alertness are induced. Tranquillizers such as the benzodiazepine derivatives may reduce the capability to perceive pain by decreasing alertness. Moreover, such tranquillizers can diminish impulse transmission in the spinal nociceptive system by increasing GABA-mediated inhibitory mechanisms (Olsen 1982) at the spinal level and reducing facilitatory influences descending from the reticular formation. A central muscle relaxant effect may help to potentiate the analgesic effect of non-steroidal anti-inflammatory drugs under conditions where a nociceptive reflex component contributes to pain sensation, as, for example, in myalgia.

Impulse transmission from primary nociceptive afferents to neurones whose axons form the spinothalamic tract is controlled by descending inhibition from the periaqueductal grey matter (PAG) and raphé nuclei (Fig. 3). Electrical stimulation

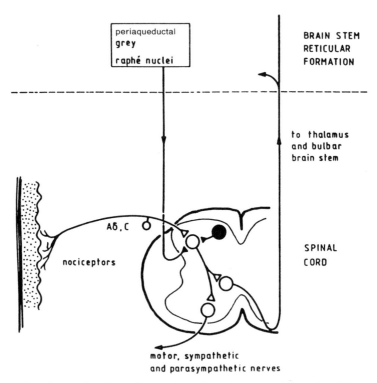

Fig. 3. Inhibition descending from the periaqueductal grey matter and raphé nuclei in the brainstem blocks impulse transmission from nociceptive afferents (see also Fig. 1).

using electrodes implanted into these brainstem areas depress nociceptive reflexes (Mayer *et al.* 1971; Reynolds 1969) and nociceptive activity in ascending axons of the spinal cord (Jurna 1980) in experiments on animals, and it may produce relief from pain in patients. Morphine activates inhibition descending from the PAG and raphé nuclei and thus inhibits nociceptive impulse transmission in the spinal cord by an action at the spinal and the supraspinal level. Descending inhibition is mediated by 5-hydroxytryptamine (Belcher *et al.* 1983; Deakin and Dostrovsky 1978; Handwerker 1976; Le Bars *et al.* 1979).

At present, the spinal mechanisms of analgesia are much better understood than the events in the brain leading to a reduced pain perception. In fact, the notion of how drugs influence pain processing at the cerebral level is mostly based on conjecture.

Since it is known that morphine and related analgesic agents produce their effects by binding to opiate receptors, regional distribution of receptor sites and accumulation of endogenous opioid peptides may serve as landmarks where typical effects of these substances are brought about.

sites of high opiate receptor density and high concentration of endogenous opioid peptides	functional significance
* substantia gelatinosa	* spinal analgesia depression of nociceptive reflexes
periaqueductal grey raphé nuclei	* descending inhibition causes spinal analgesia and depression of nociceptive reflexes
* thalamic nuclei	* depression of relaying painful messages
* striatum	* control of impulse propagation in nociceptive pathways
* limbic system	* control of emotional and effective behaviour
* hypothalamus	* control of autonomic performance and sexual behaviour

Fig. 4.

Generally, brain areas with high opiate receptor density correspond with regions containing high concentrations of endogenous opioid peptides (Atweh and Kuhar 1983; Cuello 1983) (Fig. 4). This is true for the substantia gelatinosa, where nociceptive impulse transmission can be blocked, and for the PAG and raphé nuclei, from where nociceptive impulse transmission in the spinal cord is inhibited. Large opiate receptor populations and high amounts of endogenous opioid peptides are also found in:

1. Thalamic nuclei projecting to association areas of the cerebral cortex; they play an important role in the perception of pain.

2. The striatum; it controls impulse transmission in pathways of the nociceptive system (Jurna and Heinz 1979); neuroleptic agents may produce a beneficial effect in chronic pain by acting on dopamine receptors in the nigrostriatal system.

3. The limbic system as a basis of emotional and affective behaviour; it is probably the site where morphine evokes euphoria which may become the experience leading to abuse and addiction and where antidepressant agents may act in alleviating pain.

4. The hypothalamus, where autonomic functions and sexual behaviour are influenced; sexual behaviour and pain are well known to be linked together.

The pituitary contains a remarkably high concentration of β-endorphin which is liberated into the circulation where it reaches opiate receptors in the central nervous system and the periphery. It serves as a hormone while met-enkephalin, leu-enkephalin, dynorphin, etc. are liberated as transmitters from particular neurones.

The nociceptive system is matched by an antinociceptive system which consists of all cells synthesizing and liberating endogenous opioid peptides. The antinociceptive system can be activated by various kinds of stress or manipulations such as acupuncture or transcutaneous electrical stimulation. Since complex patterns of central nervous function result from a controlled and balanced interaction of neurones releasing different neurotransmitters, it is easy to understand that the effect produced by morphine or activation of the antinociceptive system at a given site of the nociceptive system may be mimicked by drugs acting on those receptors to which the non-opioid transmitters bind.

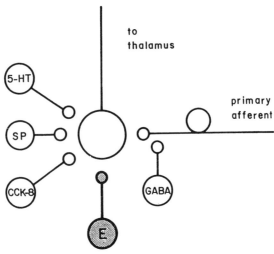

Fig. 5. *Inhibitory control of impulse transmission from nociceptive afferent (primary afferent) to the neurone sending axon to the thalamus. Inhibition is produced by the GABAergic neurone acting on the primary afferent terminal (presynaptic inhibition) or neurones releasing endorphin (E), 5-hydroxytryptamine (5-HT), substance P (SP), and cholecystokinin octapeptide (CCK-8) (postsynaptic inhibition).*

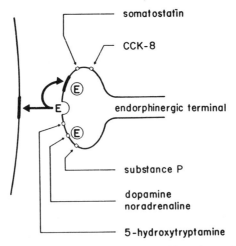

Fig. 6. *Schematic diagram showing control of endorphin release from the terminal of an endorphinergic neurone. Endorphin binds to an opiate receptor on the postsynaptic membrane and endorphinergic terminal (autoreceptor). Binding to the autoreceptor inhibits release of endorphin. Endorphin release may be enhanced by transmitters or drugs binding to respective receptors on the endorphinergic terminal (heteroreceptors). Enhanced endorphin release mimics the inhibitory effect of morphine on the postsynaptic membrane.*

Thus, for instance, impulse transmission from the terminals primary nociceptive afferents to secondary neurones is not only blocked by release of an opioid peptide from the endorphinergic neurone, but by release of 5-hydroxytryptamine, GABA, and various peptides (substance P, cholecystokinin octapeptide, and others) from the respective neurones as well (Fig. 5). In addition, the concept of presynaptic auto- and respective neurones as well (Fig. 5). In addition, the concept of presynaptic auto- and heteroreceptors permits drugs interfering with non-opiate receptor binding to produce morphine-like effects by facilitating the release of opioid peptides (Fig. 6). However, these effects of non-opioid drugs are generally limited to one or the other aspect of morphine action. In other words, and in conclusion, it may be stated that the whole range of sites of action contributing to relief of pain, i.e. from the primary afferent to highest levels of the brain, is covered only by morphine. This is the reason why morphine and related compounds are the most potent analgesic agents available.

References

Atweh, S. F. and Kuhar, M. J. (1977). Autoradiographic localization of opiate receptors in rat brain. I. Spinal cord and lower medulla. *Brain Res.* **124,** 53.
—— —— (1983). Distribution and physiological significance of opioid receptors in the brain. *Br. med. Bull.* **39,** 47.
Belcher, G., Ryall, R. W., and Schaffner, R. (1983). The differential effects of 5-hydroxytryptamine and raphé stimulation on nociceptive and non-nociceptive dorsal horn interneurones in the cat. *Brain Res.* **151,** 307.
Cuello, A. C. (1983). Central distribution of opioid peptides. *Br. med. Bull.* **39,** 11.
Deakin, J. W. F. and Dostrovsky, J. O. (1978). Involvement of the periaqueductal grey matter and spinal 5-hydroxytryptaminergic pathways in morphine analgesia: effects of lesions and 5-hydroxytryptamine depletion. *Br. J. Pharmacol.* **63,** 159.
Doi, T. and Jurna, I. (1982). Analgesic effect of intrathecal morphine demonstrated in ascending nociceptive activity in the rat spinal cord and ineffectiveness of caerulein and cholecystokinin octapeptide. *Brain Res.* **234,** 399.
Duggan, A. W., Hall, J. G., and Headley, P. M. (1977a). Enkephalins and dorsal horn neurones of the cat: effects on responses to noxious and innocuous stimuli. *Br. J. Pharmacol.* **61,** 399.
—— —— —— (1977b). Suppression of nociceptive impulses by morphine: selective effects of morphine administered in the region of the substantia gelatinosa. *Ibid.* **61,** 65.
Ferreira, S. H., Moncada, S., and Vane, J. R. (1974). Potentiation by prostaglandins of nociceptive activity of bradykinin in the dog knee joint. *Ibid.* **50,** 461P.
Fields, H. L., Emson, P. C., Leigh, B. K., Gilbert, R. F. T., and Iversen, L. L. (1980). Multiple opiate receptor sites on primary afferent fibres. *Nature, Lond.* **284,** 351.
Flower, R. J. (1974). Drugs which inhibit prostaglandin biosynthesis. *Pharmacol. Rev.* **26,** 33.
Handwerker, H. O. (1976). Influences of algogenic substances and prostaglandins on the discharges of unmyelinated cutaneous nerve fibers identified as nociceptors. In *Advances in pain research and therapy* (ed. J. J. Bonica and D. Albe-Fessard) p. 41. Raven Press, New York.
—— (1980). Pain producing substances. In *Pain and society* (ed. H. W. Kosterlitz and L. Y. Terenius) p. 325. Verlag Chemie Weinheim/Deerfield Beach, Basel.
Jurna, I. (1980). Effect of stimulation in the periaqueductal grey matter on activity in ascending axons of the rat spinal cord: selective inhibition of activity evoked by afferent $A\delta$ and C fibre stimulation and failure of naloxone to reduce inhibition. *Brain Res.* **196,** 33.
—— and Grossmann, W. (1977). The effect of morphine on mammalian nerve fibres. *Eur. J. Pharmacol.* **44,** 339.
—— and Heinz, G. (1979a). Differential effects of morphine and opioid analgesics on A and C fibre-evoked activity in ascending axons of the rat spinal cord. *Brain Res.* **171,** 573.
—— —— (1979b). Anti-nociceptive effect of morphine, opioid analgesics and haloperidol injected into the caudate nucleus of the rat. *Naunyn-Schmiedeberg's Arch. Pharmacol.* **309,** 145.

LeBars, D., Rivot, J. P., Guilbaud, G., Menétrey, D., and Besson, J. M. (1979). The depressive effect of morphine on the C fibre response of dorsal horn neurones in the spinal rat pretreated or not by pCPA. *Brain Res.* **176,** 337.

Mayer, D. J., Wofle, H., Akil, H., Carder, B., and Liebeskind, J. C. (1971). Analgesia from electrical stimulation in the brain stem of the rat. *Science, NY* **174,** 1351.

Moncada, S., Ferreira, S. H., and Vane, J. R. (1975). Inhibition of prostaglandin biosynthesis as the mechanism of analgesia of aspirine-like drugs in the knee joint. *Eur. J. Pharmacol.* **31,** 250.

Olsen, R. W. (1982). Drug interactions at the GABA receptor-ionophore complex. *Ann. Rev. Pharmacol. Toxicol.* **22,** 245.

Reynolds, D. V. (1969). Surgery in the rat during electrical analgesia induced by focal brain stimulation. *Science, NY* **164,** 444.

A brief review of postoperative pain

G. SMITH

Department of Anaesthetics
University of Leicester School of Medicine,
Leicester

It is well known that the quality of care in the management of postoperative pain is poor. In various surveys, some 40 per cent of patients complained of inadequate analgesia following minor surgery (Morrison *et al.* 1971; Keeri-Szanto and Heaman 1972). Many reasons have been proposed for this, including: delegation of management to junior surgical staff, who in turn delegate the responsibility to nursing staff; fear of inducing addiction and respiratory depression; and the failure of doctors to acknowledge a patient's distress.

Even when these factors are absent, the effective control of pain remains difficult for several reasons:

Difficulty in defining and measuring pain;
Pain variability as a result of physiological and psychological factors;
Pharmacodynamic variation to analgesic drugs accompanied by unwanted side-effects.

Pain is an extraordinarily complex sensation which may be described broadly as an integration of afferent nociceptive stimulation with interpretation of these signals by higher centres involving previous experience, memory and interpretation, and an emotive or affective component. Unfortunately, the sensation may be generated by affect itself without any obvious external stimulation. However, it is difficult to subdivide pain into physical or mental classifications and it is preferable to regard it as a spectrum comprising conscious discomfort, autonomic changes, and emotional qualities embracing fear and depression.

Most pain encountered clinically is transitory and it may be mild or severe, e.g. postoperative pain. Occasionally the pain becomes chronic and intractable. Patients with chronic pain generally present with either terminal disease or with normal life expectancy. Treatment is generally easier in the former than the latter category.

Treatment of acute pain requires attention to suppression of afferent nociceptive stimulation at either peripheral or central sites, suppression of autonomic accompaniments to painful stimuli, and therapy for the affective component. Different modes of therapy have different efficacies at these sites; the most obvious example being local anaesthetic techniques, which fall outside the remit of this article.

Advances in Morphine Therapy. The 1983 International Symposium on Pain Control, edited by E. Wilkes, 1984: Royal Society of Medicine International Congress and Symposium Series No. 64, published by the Royal Society of Medicine.

Psychological factors which influence the extent of acute pain experienced by patients include the social background, cultural beliefs, motivation, and personality of the patient. There is a good correlation between the level of anxiety and the degree of postoperative pain experienced (Parbrook et al. 1973) and also between anxiety levels and changes in pulmonary function tests (Boyle and Parbrook 1977). There is also a correlation between anxiety levels and degree of neuroticism and it has been shown that patients with higher neuroticism/scores exhibit greater pain scores after surgery (Bond 1978).

The importance of therapy for the affective component of pain is emphasized by the observation that psychotherapy reduces the requirement for postoperative analgesia (Ulert 1967) and that diazepam also reduces the requirement for postoperative analgesia (Singh et al. 1981). The importance of physiological factors in influencing the extent of pain is demonstrated by the variation in extent of perceived pain for different types of surgery. Patients experience more severe pain following thoracic and upper abdominal surgery than following lower abdominal or peripheral surgery.

Measurement of pain

Pain is an individual subjective experience, and it is extremely difficult to assess this by objective quantitative methods. Patient questionnaires are probably the most useful technique but this introduces widespread opportunity for both subject and observer bias. In order to reduce these variables to a minimum, Beecher enumerated the principles which should be incorporated in the design of studies of pain (Beecher 1959). These comprise:

1. The use of a placebo.
2. A double-blind technique. Since the placebo response is so powerful, it is important that any subliminal bias transferred from observer to patient is eliminated. In addition any subjective bias by a patient conscious of a new mode of therapy must also be eliminated.
3. A cross-over design is desirable to reduce inter-individual variation. Whilst this may be feasible for chronic pain, it is more difficult in acute pain, e.g. postoperative pain where the intensity diminishes rapidly over a 24–48-hour period.
4. The use of a reference standard. In studies of acute severe pain, it may be unethical to use a placebo and therefore comparisons should be made against a reference standard, usually i.m. morphine.

Objective methods

A variety of objective methods have been used in an attempt to measure pain. A truly objective accurate and sensitive method of quantification would be invaluable as it would eliminate the necessity for subject and observer blind designs. Unfortunately, no objective method is more sensitive than subjective assessments.

Respiratory function tests (particularly vital capacity and forced expiratory volume/ second) have been widely employed but are only useful in respect of abdominal surgery (thoracic, upper and lower abdominal surgery). In addition these tests are not truly objective but are dependent upon patient practice, experience, and motivation.

It is now known that many factors reduce postoperative vital capacity in addition to pain, e.g. pneumoperitoneum, abdominal distension, etc. In addition, the type of surgical incision has a marked effect, e.g. cholecystectomy performed through a midline incision has a much greater effect on pulmonary function than when performed through a subcostal incision (Ali and Khan 1979).

Of the pulmonary function tests available, peak expiratory flow rate appears to correlate best with subjective linear analogue scores. Vital capacity exhibited a modest correlation whilst functional residual capacity exhibited a poor correlation with linear analogue scores (Ellis *et al.* 1982; Fell *et al.* 1982).

The stress response to surgery includes increases in circulating plasma concentrations of catecholamines, glucose, and cortisol. However, complete afferent blockade does not completely suppress the cortisol response (Moller *et al.* 1982). Measurements of urinary excretion of catecholamines have been shown to be of little value in assessing pain in patients with chronic rheumatoid arthritis (Huskisson 1974*b*). More recently, it has been demonstrated that increases in plasma adrenaline and noradrenaline concentrations after surgery correlate poorly with either linear analogue scores or respiratory function testing (Fell *et al.* 1982).

Overall, it would appear that biochemical measurements are not sufficiently specific or sensitive to be valuable in quantifying the extent of pain experienced by patients.

Subjective methods

Despite the obvious difficulty of subjective scoring of pain, these methods have the merit of assessing the total component of pain (i.e. what the patient appreciates) whereas many of the more objective methods assess only one component (e.g. the autonomic or hypothalamic component as in measurement of heart rate and arterial pressure for the former and plasma ACTH or growth hormone for the latter).

Subjective assessments must be reproducible and sensitive. Two modes of testing are commonly employed, the verbal rating scale and the numerical rating scale.

With verbal rating scales, the patient is asked to describe pain in qualitative adjectival terms, e.g. no pain, mild, moderate, severe pain. However, this possesses only four discriminant points.

These verbal rating scales correlate well with numerical rating scales although the latter possess the advantage of greatly increasing the discrimination or sensitivity. The most commonly used scale is the Linear Analogue Score which permits the patient to use an infinite number of points on a line 0 to 10 cm in length. An increase in score correlates well with increasing dilatation of the cervix (which presumably reflects an increase in the extent of pain—Rosen 1977). Recall of pain was shown to be extremely reliable (Revill *et al.* 1976).

It has been shown that patients tend to cluster their scores on a linear analogue line (Huskisson 1974*a*) and this is particularly true of children. Other disadvantages of this system are that it is difficult for elderly or very young or unintelligent patients to cooperate and also for those patients who are sedated heavily with analgesic drugs.

Acute pain is usually a transient and diminishing experience. Many investigators have used a linear analogue score applied 24 hours after surgery to assess the total quantum of pain over the preceding 24 hours. This assessment is clearly open to error in terms of subject memory (in view of the use of analgesic drugs with sedative and amnesic properties) and it is preferable to assess pain at frequent intervals, say hourly, and summate total pain scores. Alternatively, the pain intensity differences may be summed (SPID). Recently electronic techniques have been developed and this greatly facilitates the hourly assessment of pain scores on a 10 cm linear analogue line.

The Magill Pain Questionnaire (MPQ) was introduced by Melzack in 1975 to evaluate the multifaceted nature of pain. A series of adjectives is applied to assess intensity of pain, degree of affect by reference to autonomic function and fear, and interpretive aspects of pain by reference to the temporal and spatial nature of the pain. Since the time taken to complete the questionnaire is 10–20 minutes it is unsuitable for rapidly changing situations such as following the course of postoperative pain (Murrin and Rosen 1984).

Variability in response to analgesics

There are enormous pharmacokinetic and pharmacodynamic variations in response to the opioids.

Recent studies with a standard dose of pethidine demonstrated a two- to fivefold difference in peak plasma concentrations and a three- to sevenfold difference in the rate of achieving peak plasma concentrations following intramuscular injection. Plasma concentrations of the drug did not correlate with body weight or lean body mass and the greatest variation occurred following the first postoperative injection (Austin et al. 1980).

Where more steady-state plasma concentrations of drug have been attained, following the use of patient-demand systems, wide variations in requirement of analgesics are evident in comparison with intramuscular injections. With self-administered pethidine the consumption varied from 13 to 44 mg per hour (Tamsen et al. 1979). With fentanyl, the self-administered dose varied from approximately 30 µg per hour to 100 µg per hour after major peripheral vascular disease (White et al. 1979). With morphine, consumption varied from 0.3 to 9 mg per hour (Dodson 1982). A 14-fold variation was found between patients for buprenorphine (Chakravarty et al. 1979).

Side-effects of the opioids

A major reason for inadequate analgesia achieved by the conventional regimen is withholding of drug for fear of producing unwanted side-effects. This is reflected by the relatively low dosage of analgesic reported in some studies.

There is no doubt that the fear of inducing both addiction and respiratory depression is exaggerated. The former has never been seriously considered a problem by clinicians experienced in the management of postoperative pain. With regard to respiratory depression, it has been shown that in patients having upper abdominal surgery, morphine 10 mg on a fixed four-hourly regimen was not associated with any significant change in PCO_2 after surgery in comparison with the preoperative value. None the less, respiratory depression is the major limiting factor which prevents the administration of sufficiently large amounts of drug to guarantee analgesia. With continuous i.v. papaveretum, in a dose judged by a patient's response to an initial bolus i.v. dose, signs of respiratory depression and potentially life threatening changes in a respiratory pattern have been demonstrated (Catling et al. 1980).

Other side-effects of the analgesic drugs include hypotension, nausea, dryness of mouth, undue sedation, and rashes (Church 1979), although these are not as limiting as respiratory depression.

Differing modes of administration of opioids

There are eight methods by which analgesics may be administered:
(i) orally; (ii) sublingually; (iii) by intramuscular injection 'on demand'—the conventional regimen; (iv) by regular i.m. injection; (v) by continuous i.v. infusion; (vi) by patient regulated i.v. injection with or without a low background infusion; (vii) rectally; and (viii) by extradural or subarachnoid injection.

The oral route for morphine and the sublingual route for buprenorphine have been employed recently with similar degrees of efficacy as conventional i.m. morphine (Ellis et al. 1982; Fell et al. 1982), but these routes, in addition to the rectal route for the administration of hydrogel-morphine (Hanning et al. 1982) and the extradural/subarachnoid routes will not be considered further.

Conventional i.m. morphine 'on demand' in a standard dose is clearly an inappropriate mode of therapy for reasons which have already been outlined—notably it fails to take into account inter- and intra-individual differences in drug requirements and variations in pain intensity in a single individual over a short period, together with variation in drug absorption from an i.m. injection (Austin et al. 1980).

These problems are obviated by the use of continuous i.v. infusions of drug. This has been shown to produce good pain relief (Church 1979; Stapleton et al. 1979; Catling et al. 1980), but carried the risk of inducing respiratory depression (Catling et al. 1980; Church 1979). Furthermore, analgesia may be obtained with lower peak concentrations of drug than those following i.m. injection (Nayman 1979). In addition, some of these studies demonstrated apparently minimum effective plasma concentrations required for analgesia—0.46 μg/ml for pethidine (Stapleton et al. 1979) and 23–25 ng/ml for morphine (Nayman 1979).

Possibly as a result of the lower peak concentrations of analgesic achieved with continuous i.v. infusions of morphine, this technique is accompanied by reported fewer side-effects than following i.m. injection (Nayman 1979).

A method of reducing but not eliminating the extent of respiratory depression inherent in the use of continuous i.v. infusions, is for the patient himself to regulate the dosage of i.v. drug. Several such systems have been described (Evans et al. 1976; Keeri-Szanto 1980; Bennett et al. 1982). A more sophisticated device is the Newcastle interactive palliator, in which a continuous low-dose i.v. infusion is combined with a patient-operated demand increment (White et al. 1979).

The disadvantage of these devices is that currently they are all bulky and expensive and the danger of respiratory depression, although lower than that with continuous i.v. infusions, is not entirely eliminated. In general, the use of these machines has been associated with production of good analgesia.

Recently, however, it has been shown in a double-blind controlled trial that patient self-administered fentanyl fails to produce superior analgesia than a control group of patients receiving regular intramuscular morphine (Welchew 1982). This is surprising in view of the theoretical advantages possessed by patient-operated on-demand analgesic computers (notably the production of more constant plasma concentrations of opioid and a more ostensible placebo effect) and this may reflect the insensitive techniques currently available for the measurement of pain.

References

Ali, J. and Khan, T. A. (1979). The comparative effects of muscle transection and median upper abdominal incisions on postoperative pulmonary function. *Surg. Gynecol. Obstet.* **148**, 863.

Austin, K. L., Stapleton, J. V., and Mather, L. E. (1980). Multiple intramuscular injections: a major source of variability in analgesic response to meperidine. *Pain* **8**, 47.

Beecher, H. K. (1959). *Measurement of subjective responses.* Oxford University Press, New York.

Bennett, R. L., Batenhurst, R. L., Bivins, B. A., Bell, R. M., Graves, D. A., Foster, T. S., Wright, B. D., and Griffin, W. O. (1982). Patient controlled analgesia. *Annals Surg.* **195**, 700.

Bond, M. R. (1978). Psychological and psychiatric aspects of pain. *Anaesthesia* **33**, 355.

Boyle, P. and Parbrook, G. D. (1977). The inter-relation of personality and postoperative factors. *Br. J. Anaesth.* **49**, 259.

Catling, J. A., Pinto, D. M., Jordan, C., and Jones, J. G. (1980). Respiratory effects of analgesics after cholecystectomy: comparison of continuous oral intermittent papaveretum. *Br. med. J.* **281**, 478.

Chakravarty, K., Tucker, W., Rosen, M., and Vickers, M. D. (1979). Comparison of buprenorphine and pethidine given intravenously on demand to relieve postoperative pain. *Br. med. J.* **ii**, 895.

Church, J. J. (1979). Continuous narcotic infusions for relief of postoperative pain. *Br. med. J.* **i**, 977.

Dodson, M. (1982). A review of methods for relief of postoperative pain. *Annals R. Coll. Surg.* **64**, 324.

Ellis R., Haines, D., Shah, R., Cotton, B. R., and Smith, G. (1982). Pain relief after abdominal surgery—a comparison of i.m. morphine, sublingual buprenorphine and self-administered i.v. pethidine. *Br. J. Anaesth.* **54**, 421.

Evans, J. M., Rosen, M., McCarthy, J., and Hogg, M. I. J. (1976). Apparatus for patient-controlled administration of intravenous narcotics during labour. *Lancet* **i**, 17.

Fell, D., Chmielewski, A., and Smith, G. (1982). Postoperative analgesia with controlled release morphine sulphate. *Br. med. J.* **285**, 92.

Hanning, C. D., Smith, G., McNeill, M., and Graham, N. B. (1983). Rectal administration of morphine from a sustained release hydrogel suppository. *Br. J. Anaesth.* **55**, (3) 236P–237P (Abstract).

Huskisson, E. C. (1974a). Measurement of pain. *Lancet* **ii**, 1127.

—— (1974b). Catecholamine excretion and pain. *Br. J. clin. Pharmacol.* **1**, 80.

Keeri-Szanto, M. (1980). Demand analgesia. In *Trends in intravenous analgesia* (ed. J. A. Aldrete and T. H. Stanley) Year Book Medical Publishers, Chicago.

—— and Heaman, S. (1972). Postoperative demand analgesia. *Surg. Gynecol. Obstet.* **134**, 641.

Melzack, R. (1975). The Magill Pain Questionnaire: major properties and scoring methods. *Pain* **1**, 277.

Moller, I. W., Rem, J., Brandt, M. R., and Kehlet, H. (1982). Effect of post-traumatic epidural analgesia on the cortisol and hyperglycaemic response to surgery. *Acta anaesth. scand.* **26**, 56.

Morrison, J. D., Loan, W. B., and Dundee, J. W. (1971). Controlled comparison of the efficacy of 14 preparations in the relief of postoperative pain. *Br. med. J.* **iii**, 287.

Murrin, K. R. and Rosen, M. (1984). The measurement of pain. In *Acute pain* (ed. G. Smith and B. Covino). Butterworths, London.

Nayman, J. (1979). Measurement and control of postoperative pain. *Annals R. Coll. Surg.* **61**, 419.

Parbrook, G. D., Steel, D. F., and Dalrymple, D. G. (1973). Factors predisposing to postoperative pain and pulmonary complications. A study of male patients undergoing elective gastric surgery. *Br. J. Anaesth.* **45**, 21.

Revill, S. I., Robinson, J. O., Rosen, M., and Hogg, M. I. J. (1976). The reliability of a linear analogue for evaluating pain. *Anaesthesia* **31,** 1191.

Rosen, M. (1977). The measurement of pain. In *Pain. New perspectives in measurement and management* (ed. A. W. Harcus, R. Smith, and B. Whittle). Churchill Livingstone, London.

Singh, P. N., Sharma, P., Gupta, P. K., and Pandey, K. (1981). Clinical evaluation of diazepam for relief of postoperative pain. *Br. J. Anaesth.* **53,** 831.

Stapleton, J. V., Austin, K. L., and Mather, L. E. (1979). A pharmacokinetic approach to postoperative pain: continuous infusion of pethidine. *Anaesth. Intens. Care* **7,** 25.

Tamsen, A., Hartvig, P., Dahlström, B., Lindström, B., and Holmdahl, M. (1979). Patient controlled analgesic therapy in the early postoperative period. *Acta anaesth. scand.* **23,** 462.

Ulert, I. A. (1967). Narcotics in the postoperative period: a reappraisal. *South. med. J.* **60,** 1289.

Welchew, E. A. (1982). A postoperative pain recorder. A patient-controlled recording device for assessing postoperative pain. *Anaesthesia* **37,** 838.

White, W. D., Pearce, D. J., and Norman, J. (1979). Postoperative analgesia: a comparison of intravenous on-demand fentanyl with epidural bupivacaine. *Br. med. J.* **ii,** 166.

A comparison of the effects on gastric emptying of the route of administration of morphine

G. R. PARK, BSc., MB, ChB., FFARCS

Lecturer in Anaesthesia,
Department of Anaesthetics,
Royal Infirmary,
Edinburgh

Present appointment:
Consultant in Anaesthesia and Intensive Care,
Addenbrooke's Hospital,
Hills Road,
Cambridge

D. WEIR, MB., ChB.

Registrar,
Department of Anaesthetics,
Royal Infirmary,
Edinburgh

Abstract

A new long-acting oral preparation (OCR) of morphine (MST Continus tablets, Napp Laboratories Ltd.) can give analgesia as good as that provided by the conventional use of intramuscular morphine following hysterectomy and cholecystectomy (Fell *et al.* 1982). It was also noted that more sedation occurred following oral morphine. These properties of long-acting analgesia (Leslie *et al.* 1980) and sedation make it attractive for use as a premedicant prior to certain types of surgery. Before a drug is used in this manner it is important to ensure that no adverse effects exist which might increase the risk of anaesthesia. Oral morphine-like substances are used for decreasing gastro-intestinal mobility. The effect of oral morphine on gastric emptying might be important, if delay does occur this might increase the risk of vomiting and subsequent aspiration of stomach contents into the lung. We have therefore compared the effects

Advances in Morphine Therapy. The 1983 International Symposium on Pain Control, edited by E. Wilkes, 1984: Royal Society of Medicine International Congress and Symposium Series No. 64, published by the Royal Society of Medicine.

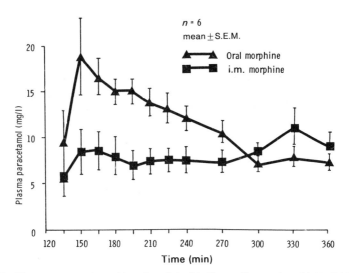

Fig. 1. Plasma paracetamol levels related to time after oral and i.m. morphine.

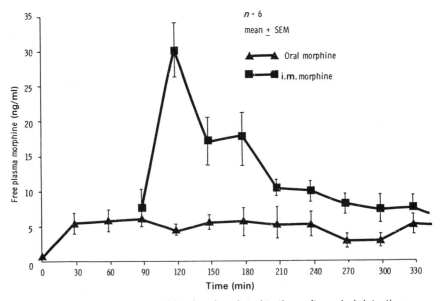

Fig. 2. Free plasma morphine levels related to time after administration.

of 20 mg oral controlled-release morphine and a conventional premedicant dose of 10 mg morphine intramuscularly using paracetamol absorption as an indicator of gastric emptying. Absorption of paracetamol occurs from the small intestine and not from the stomach, if gastric emptying is delayed then paracetamol will be absorbed slowly which will be reflected by low plasma levels. The study was approved by the hospital ethical committee.

Six healthy male volunteers were studied on two occasions at least one week apart. On one occasion they received 20 mg OCR morphine at time 0 min, and on the other

10 mg morphine intramuscularly at 90 min. Paracetamol 1500 mg in orange squash was administered orally at 120 min. Venous blood was sampled for both paracetamol and morphine levels during the study.

The overall mean plasma paracetamol level was higher following OCR morphine (11.4 mg/l : 7.45 mg/l OCR/i.m.) as was the peak paracetamol level (Fig. 1) which was only slightly lower than that seen in volunteers who have received placebos (Heading *et al.* 1973). Free plasma morphine levels were lower following OCR morphine than i.m. morphine and did not reach its peak value for 90 min (7.33 ± 2.08 ng/ml). Following i.m. morphine peak values were reached in 30 min and were much higher (30.58 ± 4.10 ng/ml) (Fig. 2). The fourfold difference has been described previously (Brunk and Delle 1974).

It would appear that the administration of 20 mg OCR morphine does not delay gastric emptying significantly. Further studies on its use preoperatively appear to be indicated.

References

Brunk, S. F. and Delle, M. (1974). Morphine metabolism in man. *Clin. Pharmacol. Ther.* **1**, 51–7.

Fell, D., Chmielewski, A. M., and Smith, G. (1982). Post operative analgesia with controlled release morphine sulphate: comparison with intramuscular morphine. *Br. med. J.* **285**, 92–4.

Heading, R. C., Nimmo, J., Prescott, L. F., and Tothill, P. (1973). The dependence of paracetamol absorbtion on the rate of gastric emptying. *Br. J. Pharmacol.* **47**, 415–21.

Leslie, S. T., Rhodes, A., and Black, F. M. (1980). Controlled-release morphine sulphate tablets—a study in normal volunteers. *Br. J. clin. Pharmacol.* **9**, 531–4.

Premedication of children using morphine sulphate Continus tablets

E. G. HADAWAY

Kettering and District General Hospital

Summary

Morphine sulphate Continus tablets (MST Continus tablets, Napp Laboratories Ltd.) were used in a dose of 1 mg/kg body weight for the premedication of children aged 4–12 years, undergoing elective tonsillectomy. The morphine was well absorbed and high plasma morphine concentrations were recorded between 180 and 340 minutes after administration.

Compared with papaveretum 0.3 mg/kg body weight given intramuscularly 100 minutes preoperatively to a control group, the tablets were more acceptable to the patients, though not significantly. Preoperative vomiting was significantly more frequent in the oral group, but there were no significant differences in preoperative sedation, recovery time, postoperative vomiting or requirements for postoperative analgesia. Neither group suffered any serious problems attributable to morphine.

It is concluded that morphine sulphate Continus tablets are useful for premedication in children having elective surgery. It is suggested that an antiemetic be included in the premedication.

A trial of premedication for children was undertaken to investigate the following aspects of morphine sulphate Continus tablets:

1. Acceptability of the oral route.
2. Duration of action as evidenced by:
    (a) behaviour at different intervals after administration;
    (b) plasma morphine concentrations at the time of operation;
    (c) requirements for postoperative analgesia.
3. Any undesirable effects.

Patients and methods

Patients admitted to the trial were aged 4–12 years and were to undergo elective tonsillectomy. All were admitted the day before the operation and all operations took place in the morning.

Advances in Morphine Therapy. The 1983 International Symposium on Pain Control, edited by E. Wilkes, 1984: Royal Society of Medicine International Congress and Symposium Series No. 64, published by the Royal Society of Medicine.

Patients who were obviously unco-operative owing to mental subnormality; those with severe cardiorespiratory, hepatic or renal disease; and those receiving drugs likely to influence the effects of opiates or anaesthetics were excluded from the trial.

The patients were randomly assigned to two groups.

Group A—66 patients

Patients in Group A were prescribed papaveretum 0.3 mg/kg body weight injected intramuscularly one hour preoperatively.

Group B—67 patients

Patients in Group B were prescribed morphine sulphate Continus tablets in a dose of 1 mg/kg body weight at 06.00 hours regardless of the expected time of operation. Since the smallest tablets were 10 mg and it was thought that excessive division of the tablets might affect the rate of absorption, fractions of less than one-half of a tablet were not used and the dosage was, therefore rounded down to the nearest 5 mg. Tablets were divided when necessary with a knife and were swallowed without crushing or chewing.

A standard anaesthetic technique was followed for all patients. Anaesthesia was induced with thiopentone 2.5 per cent intravenously, 4 mg/kg body weight on the dorsum of the hand using an intravenous needle size 25. This was followed by suxamethonium 1 mg/kg body weight. Intubation was with an uncuffed oral endotracheal tube and anaesthesia was maintained with nitrous oxide, oxygen, and halothane. Respiration was spontaneous. Droperidol 0.1 mg/kg body weight was injected intramuscularly during anaesthesia as an antiemetic. Five millilitres of venous blood was taken for morphine estimation during surgery. For postoperative analgesia, papaveretum 0.3 mg/kg body weight was prescribed to be given if required intramuscularly.

Observations

A separate record card was kept for observations; it was filled in by staff who were unaware of the nature of the premedication.

Table 1 lists the observations.

Results

Groups A and B were comparable with respect to age, weight, and duration of anaesthesia. Comparisons are shown in Table 2. The results were compared using the chi-squared test with Yates' correction.

A statistically significant difference was found in the incidence of preoperative vomiting ($p = < 0.01$). There appeared to be more satisfactory behaviour in the recovery room and ward in the oral group, but neither this nor any of the other comparisons were statistically significant.

Table 1

Observations

Preoperative vomiting	— + or —
Reaction to premedication	— accept/reluctant/refuse
Behaviour in the ward preoperatively	— calm/treatful/restless/violent
State of consciousness before induction of anaesthesia	— asleep/awake and calm/restless/violent
Reaction to intravenous injection	— nil/winced/restless/violent
Time of induction of anaesthesia	—
Time of end of operation	—
Anaesthetic details with any comments	—
Time of blood sample	—
Time of opening eyes in recovery on verbal instruction only	—
Behaviour in recovery	— calm/tearful/restless/violent
Vomiting in recovery	— Nausea or vomit/no nausea or vomit
Analgesic given in recovery room	— + or —
Respiratory problem in recovery room	— + or — with details
Behaviour in the ward postoperatively until 18.00 h	— asleep/awake and comfortable/distressed
Vomiting in the ward postoperatively until 18.00 h	— no nausea or vomiting/nausea or vomiting
Respiratory problems in the ward postoperatively until 18.00 h	—
Analgesia given in the ward postoperatively until 18.00 h	— + or —

Morphine measurements

Plasma morphine concentrations were measured by radioimmunoassay using a [^{125}I]-morphine label prepared by the Nuffield Department of Clinical Biochemistry, Oxford and a specific antiserum. The least amount of morphine measurable was 0.5 ng/ml of plasma. Coefficients of variation for control samples were less than 10 per cent for values between 10 and 100 ng/ml. The comparative concentrations at the time of operation were in ng/ml of plasma.

    Group A — Mean   50.3 SD 22.8   — Median 49.
    Group B — Mean   137.8 SD 92   — Median 125.

This difference was highly significant using the median test $p \ll 0.05$. Figures 1 and 2 relate plasma morphine concentrations to the interval between administration and

Table 2

Comparisons of Groups A and B

	Group A		Group B	
Mean age (nearest birthday)	6.85	SD 2.17	6.84	SD 1.87
Mean body weight (kg)	23.5	SD 7.1	23.6	SD 8.5
Mean duration of anaesthetic (min)	28.2	SD 8.2	28.9	SD 8.2
Acceptability				
Accepted	50		57	
Reluctant/refused	16		9	
Preoperative vomiting				
No vomit	64		51	
Vomit	2		16	
Behaviour preoperatively				
Satisfactory—calm	54		51	
Unsatisfactory—tearful/restless/violent	11		10	
Consciousness in the anaesthetic room				
Satisfactory—asleep/calm	56		58	
Unsatisfactory—restless	9		8	
Reaction to injection				
Satisfactory—nil	30		36	
Unsatisfactory—wince/restless/violent	34		28	
Median recovery time (min)	20		23	
Mean recovery time (min)	21	SD 8.8	23	SD 11.4
Analgesics in recovery room				
Given—	26		21	
Not given—	40		45	
Behaviour in recovery				
Calm—	15		23	
Unsatisfactory: tearful/restless/violent	51		43	
Vomiting in recovery				
Nausea or vomit	3		8	
No nausea or vomit	62		58	
Respiratory problems in recovery				
Possibly attributable to morphine	1 (breath holding)		1 (cyanosis—details not stated)	
Behaviour in the ward postoperatively				
Satisfactory—asleep/comfortable	52		59	
Unsatisfactory—distressed	12		7	
Vomiting in the ward postoperatively				
Nausea or vomiting	26		26	
No nausea or vomiting	39		40	
Respiratory problems in the ward possibly attributable to morphine	0		1 (shallow breathing—no treatment required)	
Postoperative analgesia in the ward				
Given	4		5	
Not given	61		61	

There were no serious respiratory problems in either group attributable to morphine.

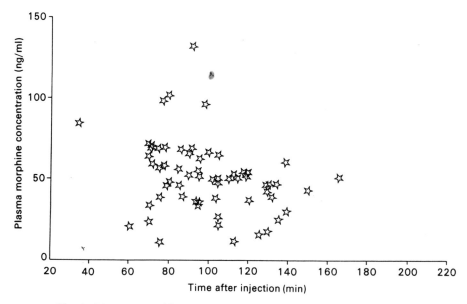

Fig. 1. Plasma morphine concentration related to time after injection.

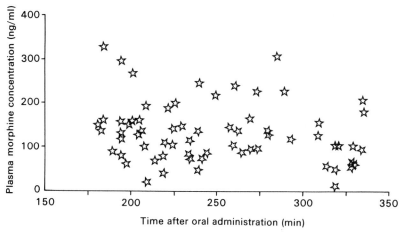

Fig. 2. Plasma morphine concentration related to time after oral administration.

operation. There was no obvious relationship between the concentration and the interval in either group.

The oral group was divided into high and low concentration groups, i.e. those up to and including the median level of 125 ng/ml and those above this figure. These two groups were compared as shown in Table 3.

Discussion

Morphine sulphate Continus tablets are intended for the treatment of chronic pain (Twycross 1981). Although it has been claimed that they are not useful in acute pain

Table 3

Percentages of 'satisfactory' patients in 'high' and 'low' oral groups

	Low group	High group
1. No nausea or vomiting		
(a) Preoperative	82	79
(b) Postoperative in the recovery room	82	94
(c) Postoperative on the ward	67	54
2. Satisfactory preoperative behaviour	90	78
3. Satisfactory consciousness in the anaesthetic room	91	84
4. No reaction to intravenous injection	53	59
5. Satisfactory behaviour in the recovery room	33	34
6. No analgesic requirements in the recovery room	67	69
7. Satisfactory behaviour in the ward postoperatively	91	88
8. No analgesic requirements in the ward postoperatively	91	94
9. Recovery time		
Mean	20.3 SD 11.3	24.9 SD 11.2
Median	18.5	25.5

There were no statistically significant differences between the 'high' and 'low' groups in any of these comparisons.

(*Drugs and Therapeutics Bulletin* 1981) they have been used with success postoperatively (Fell *et al.* 1982).

As yet, the use of morphine sulphate Continus tablets in children has not been investigated.

Oral premedication is generally considered to be less distressing for children than intramuscular injection. The most popular oral premedication for children is probably still trimeprazine tartrate syrup, despite its long-recognized lack of analgesic and euphoriant actions (Davis and Doughty 1966). A long-acting oral morphine preparation might be expected to produce euphoria and analgesia to facilitate intravenous induction of anaesthesia, while being more acceptable to the patient than an intramuscular injection. In fact the tablets were preferred, but not significantly.

It was thought that a long-acting preparation might obviate careful timing of administration as well as reducing postoperative analgesic requirements. The ward staff considered that giving tablets at a standard time was easier than attempting to estimate the correct time for injections. It is noted that the mean time for intramuscular premedication was actually 101 minutes compared with the 60 minutes desired.

The plasma morphine concentrations shown in Figs. 1 and 2 show a wide variation. Therapeutic concentrations (Dunnill *et al.* 1979) persisted after five hours in 13 out of 14 patients in the oral group, while the effects of intramuscular morphine would be expected to be waning after this interval. The controlled-release characteristic of the tablets is therefore of value in this respect. However, surprisingly there was no significant reduction in postoperative analgesic requirements or improvement in postoperative behaviour in the oral group.

The dosage of 1 mg/kg body weight had been clinically satisfactory in preliminary use over approximately one year, and was therefore compared with a commonly used dose of 0.3 mg/kg of intramuscular papaveretum. It has been suggested that the relative dose of oral to intramuscular morphine should be about 2:1 (Fell *et al.* 1982). However, using approximately three times the dose the median morphine concentration was 125 ng/ml, with the controlled-release oral preparation compared with 49 ng/ml in the intramuscular group. Absorption of the oral preparation was, therefore, higher than predicted. The mean time after the intramuscular dose was 101 minutes at which time a high level might be expected. However, the mean time after administration of the oral group was 248 minutes and a relatively steady level might be predicted (Leslie *et al.* 1980). The high levels of morphine in the oral group were interesting in that they were not related to the degree of sedation. Indeed the highest figure of 639 ng/ml of plasma was in a patient who was not heavily sedated. Recovery time was little affected by the plasma morphine concentration. Even the 'high' oral group had a mean recovery time of 24.9 minutes compared with 21 minutes in the intramuscular group. Thus, plasma levels reflect absorption rather than sedation. The therapeutic range of plasma morphine concentration has been put at 50–500 ng/ml, a typical peak after normal intramuscular dosage being 70 ng/ml (Dunnill *et al.* 1979). Figures obtained in this trial fall mainly within this range.

Vomiting was a greater problem preoperatively after the oral premedication than after intramuscular injection. It was not possible clearly to identify patients who were particularly likely to vomit preoperatively. However, it was noted that of preoperative vomits, all except one occurred in children aged six, seven, and eight years. These comprised 55 per cent of the patients in the trial. There was no evident relationship between plasma morphine concentrations and the incidence of vomiting. Postoperatively there was little difference between groups even after the relatively low intramuscular dose of 0.1 mg/kg of droperidol. Therefore an antiemetic is desirable with morphine sulphate Continus tablets and the author is currently adding droperidol syrup 0.3 mg/kg to the premedication regimen.

The lack of respiratory problems which could be attributable to morphine, indicates that morphine is a safe drug using these doses, for relatively fit children.

Acknowledgements

Thanks are due to the following: Napp Laboratories Ltd. for the supply of materials and help with organization of the trial; Dr P. Treasure of the Department of Community Medicine, The University of Cambridge, for statistical analysis; Dr R. A. Moore, Principal Biochemist, The Nuffield Department of Clinical Biochemistry, Oxford, for measuring plasma morphine concentrations; Mr J. R. Page and Mr R. T. J. Shortridge, Kettering General Hospital, for permission to study their patients; and the nursing, secretarial, and junior anaesthetic staff at Kettering General Hospital, for their co-operation in the trial.

References

Davis, D. R. and Doughty, A. (1966). Oral premedication in children with trimeprazine. *Br. J. Anaesth.* **38,** 878.

Drug and Therapeutics Bulletin (1981). Morphine in slow-release tablets. *Drug Ther. Bull.* **19,** 11.

Dunnill, R. P. H., Colvin, M. P., and Crawley, B. E. (1979). *Clinical resuscitative data*, 2nd ed. Blackwell, Oxford.

Fell, D., Chmielewski, A., and Smith, G. (1982). Post-operative analgesia with controlled-release morphine sulphate: comparison with intramuscular morphine. *Br. med. J.* **285,** 92.

Leslie, S. T., Rhodes, A., and Black, F. M. (1980). Controlled-release morphine sulphate tablets—a study in normal volunteers. *Br. J. clin. Pharmacol.* **9,** 531.

Twycross, R. G. (1981). Controlled release morphine tablets. *Lancet* **i,** 892.

Postoperative pain therapy in neurosurgery and orthopaedics in patients suffering from chronic pain at the Mainz Pain Centre

H. U. GERBERSHAGEN

Schmerz-Zentrum Mainz,
Mainz

The Mainz Pain Centre only takes in patients suffering from chronic pain. The team of doctors, psychologists, social workers, and nurses regards the treatment of acute pain as a problem which can be solved. This opinion is contrary to the opinion of many hundreds of publications concerning postoperative pain control which are available on our own computer system or in international medical data storage units.

Optimum postoperative supervision and care, which always includes a preoperative explanation to the patient and information about the probable postoperative outcome, will not only consist of tender loving care, but also of professionalism. Here too, the patient's rights and duties must be taken into account. It is certainly the patient's right to suffer a minimum of moderate to severe pain after an operation. It is the patient's duty—according to our leisurely preoperative explanation—to make pain relief possible. That is to say, it is the patient's duty to report the onset of pain (or as the dictum has it: 'in the postoperative period, heroism is neither required nor beneficial to the healing process'). This attitude, that the patient has the right to expect or to demand satisfactory postoperative pain relief, is generally unknown to doctors, nursing staff, and patients. If, for a change, doctors become patients and undergo surgery, this right is often eloquently cited; whole editorials and leading articles get written. These usually draw attention to the current lack of medical knowledge relating to the pharmacokinetics and pharmacology of analgesics and psychopharmacological drugs, to the psychology of patients suffering from acute pain, and to the personality structure of those suffering from chronic pain. The doctors' fear of prescribing and the nurses' fear of administering or injecting adequate doses of pain-killers at adequate intervals appears to me—quite apart from the ideological education or cultural origins of the team of doctors responsible—to be the main motive for unsatisfactory postoperative pain control. Assertions that approximately 90 per cent of postoperative pain can be controlled by placebo support the prescription of ineffective doses of analgesics.

Advances in Morphine Therapy. The 1983 International Symposium on Pain Control, edited by E. Wilkes, 1984: Royal Society of Medicine International Congress and Symposium Series No. 64, published by the Royal Society of Medicine.

As doctors, we must analyse the factors which constitute the extent of the measures necessary for combatting postoperative pain. For decades, attention has repeatedly been drawn to the importance of:

1. *The location of surgical intervention* as a quantity which can be readily determined.

2. *The extent and duration of surgery* (often without taking into account the trauma caused by anaesthesia which invariably persists for some time).

3. *The time which has elapsed since operation* (pain killers are *seldom* requested on the third postoperative day).

4. *The patient's personality structure is constantly cited* (often it has only been superficially determined using various psychometric tests; often without in-depth knowledge of psychology on the part of those making the diagnosis and those giving the treatment).

Table 1

	Rotator cuff repair and AC-joint resection	Lumbar fusion (bone graft from iliac crest	Laminectomy, facetectomy lesions	Dorsal root entry zone
Number of body complaints	34.2 ± 9.1	37.4 ± 10.7	31.7 ± 9.6	29.1 ± 16.3
Number of psychological complaints	25.4 ± 12.3	32.8 ± 13.4	28.6 ± 9.3	29.8 ± 13.2
Number of pain descriptors	16.0 ± 10.3	23.8 ± 19.4	25.8 ± 17.0	36.8 ± 33.6

Essential factors, such as careful, tissue-conserving operating techniques and the administration of adapted anaesthesia are not included for various reasons. On the other hand, possible differences are pointed out between surgical wards (Table 1). The fact is obscured that the doctor is responsible for the patient and that the nursing staff will be proud of the doctor who prescribes sensible, comprehensible measures for pain relief. The often quoted reference to special institutions and different wards having their own traditions and practices is understandable; however, the patient has the right to adequate pain relief.

In my opinion, there is only one exception to non-a priori completely satisfactory pain medication: the situation in which studies are being made of analgesics. The testing of analgesics is carried out in serious institutions according to international standards and in accordance with the Helsinki Declaration. Only these patients take the calculable risk, from which they can withdraw at any time, of severe postoperative pain.

However, if one looks at the large number of studies published on analgesics, it is conspicuous that in the majority of studies the patients were given the test drug at the start of moderate (and often slight) pain. The value of these studies for the use of powerful analgesics should accordingly be assessed critically by the medical profession—not logically by the individual Regional Health Authorities.

The requirements to be fulfilled by ideal analgesics are often quoted. These utopian estimations must act as maxims for the research laboratories, but for the clinician they are often the inducement to undersupply the patient suffering from postoperative pain.

Table 2

	Rotator cuff repair and AC-joint resection (n = 25)	Lumbar fusions (n = 25)	Laminectomy and facetectomy (n = 25)	Dorsal root entry zone lesions (n = 25)
Age (years)	53.6±11.6	43.4±7.6	50.2±8.7	50.4±13.3
Sex distribution	18 F:7 M	21 F:4 M	15 F:10 M	5 F:20 M
Weight (kg)	70.4±13.5	70.5±11.6	75.4±13.7	67.7±11.5
Height (cm)	165.3±7.0	168.6±7.9	171.6±9.9	170.5±8.6
ASA anaesthetik risk I II III	6 18 1	2 17 6	2 23 –	2 14 9
Anaesthesia	E/F = 25	E/F = 22; NLA = 3	E/F = 21; NLA = 4	E/F = 16, NLA = 9
Duration of anaesthesia (min)	61.2±20.6	160±30.7	172.9±66.4	336.6±65.7
Duration of surgery (min)	25.6±10.8	113.5±24.8	112.5±40.3	274.1±59.9
Hours to first analgesic	4.4±0.5	1.8±1.3	3.1±2.8	2.9±0.5
Injections, first 24 h	3.7±1.8	6.2±1.8	4.7±1.9	4.8±1.5
Injections, second 24 h	2.7±0.6	3.2±1.9	3.0±1.7	3.0±1.7
Pethidine (mg) first 24 h	220.2±128.1	435.4±126.3	347.4±130.7	319.6±109.0
Pethidine (mg) second 24 h	262.5±178.5 (4 pts)	230.8±178.5 (13 pts)	240.6±126.0 (8 pts)	210.4±116.5 (9 pts)
PO doses Tramadol second 24 h	2.1±1.1 (10 pts)	4.8±2.0 (10 pts)	3.7±2.3 (7 pts)	3.3±1.7 (6 pts)
Tramadol (mg) second 24 h	101.0±48.4 (10 pts)	240.0±99.4 (10 pts)	185.7±114.4	131.7±69.4 (6 pts)

The drugs should take effect as soon as possible after administration. They should have a powerful action and should of course aim to provide freedom from pain lasting for many hours. The preparations should have a wide therapeutic range and negligible toxicity. The most important organ system functions (respiration, cardiac circulation, intestinal tract, urogenital system, cerebral functions) should be scarcely affected. Central side-effects such as nausea and vomiting should not occur. Local tolerability of various forms of administration and compatibility with vehicles are self-evident.

Our many years of investigations of analgesic drugs during the postoperative period have disillusioned us by showing that all currently known analgesics *when administered in equally potent dosages*—irrespective of previous drugs administered and of the patient's personality structure—achieve the same results in the relief of pain and produce the same side-effects. This opinion contradicts once again the majority of published studies. Study design and implementation should be examined critically by neutral bodies before publication.

In our centre, only those patients were operated on who had suffered pain for many years. With the exception of the group of patients with torn rotator cuffs and acromioclavicular articulation arthroses, our patients had already been operated on in the same place several times before and were familiar with the consequences and side-effects of operations. As a matter of routine, our patients were promised good postoperative pain relief; this is in any case necessary, since our patients mostly suffer from reactive or endoreactive depression.

All the patients were extubated in a wakeful and co-operative condition in the operating theatre. If narcotics were injected during anaesthesia, these were antagonized.

In order to demonstrate the factors which are important for postoperative pain treatment, I selected four groups of patients with differing locations and extents of intervention who had been anaesthetized for different lengths of time. The groups comprised (Table 2):

1. Kessel operations as modified by Waisbrod to attend to torn rotator cuffs and subacromial joint arthropathy.

2. Ventral and posterolateral spondylodeses (= fusion operations), including facetectomies, removal of slivers of bone from the pelvis, sometimes with laminectomies, and in some cases with the use of Knodt stabilizing rods.

3. Laminectomies and facetectomies in those who had had multiple previous operations.

4. Thermocoagulation of dorsal root entry zone lesions, which required broad laminectomy extending over several segments and 40–80 individual coagulation foci.

The patients, who were chosen consecutively, received pethidine injections every three hours (approx. 1 mg/kg body weight) for the first 18–24 hours postoperatively according to an adapted semi-rigid time scheme. After this, they received tramadol orally every four hours (approx. 0.7 mg/kg body weight). As previously agreed with the patient, the first dose was given on the first indication or complaint of pain.

Little attention was paid to the results of the division into groups according to risk on the lines of the American Association of Anaesthesia, since our earlier studies showed that underdosing with analgesics is often the result, and the patient suffers pain unnecessarily. The duration of anaesthesia and surgery corresponded to the scale of the operation. The ensuing tissue trauma determined, at least superficially, the time of the first analgesic injection. The number of injections required for adequate pain relief was governed during the first 24 hours by surgical trauma, with a high requirement being particularly noticeable in the spondylodesis group due mainly to pain at the place where slivers of bone were taken from the pelvic crest. The consumption of analgesics dropped rapidly as time elapsed after the operation. On the second post-operative day only 25–40 per cent of patients required 2–5 injections and a small amount of oral medication. On the third postoperative day only eight out of the 100 patients received oral analgesics sporadically.

Since the time scheme was also kept to at night, our patients suffered at most from slight or troublesome discomfort. It is true that the time scheme did not guarantee a constant level of analgesics, but it did provide a sufficiently effective one, so that for example unplanned dressing changes, investigations or other manipulations were not particularly painful.

The small number of cases per group made it impossible to take into account the factor of freedom from pain/influence of pain apart from wound pain. Approximately 60 per cent of paraplegics, amputees, and herpes zoster patients were free from their tormenting, destructive pain *immediately* after operation. Similar results were also obtained initially with spondylodesis and laminectomy patients, and there was a roughly 90 per cent improvement after the Kessel operation. Even investigations of large groups would not allow a meaningful and correct classification of these psychodynamically important factors. The current misuse of isolated personality factors and their significance for postoperative pain therapy should not lead to undersupplying patients with analgesics.

The doctor on a surgical ward must guarantee the patients' right to good pain relief. This is only possible through thorough knowledge of the operating techniques and the trauma they induce, through familiarity with the physiological and functional processes and through the study of analgesics and psychopharmacological drugs. The choice of the type of pain therapy (e.g. epidural anaesthesia with local anaesthesia or opiates, transcutaneous electric nerve stimulation or drug therapy) depends—apart from the factor of the doctor's personality structure—mainly on the location of the orthopaedic and neurosurgical intervention.

The semi-rigid time scheme for analgesic administration described here is effective. It calls for the co-operation of the doctor and the sister/nurse. The limiting factors in good postoperative pain therapy are purely and simply uncommitted and poorly educated doctors and nurses.

Pain relief following thoracotomy

DEIRDRE WATSON

Thoracic surgical unit,
East Birmingham Hospital,
Birmingham

Introduction

As in so many postoperative situations continuous relief of pain without oversedation or respiratory depression remains a rarely attained goal for the thoracic surgical patient. The patient who has undergone thoracotomy exemplifies the need for adequate and continuous relief of pain not only for the patient's comfort but to enable him to cough and co-operate fully with physiotherapy. Since the majority of thoracic surgical patients are able to eat and drink as soon as the immediate effects of the anaesthetic have worn off they are an ideal group to consider for oral analgesics and yet the majority of thoracic surgeons still use intramuscular opiates as their main weapon in pain control.

Materials and methods

Objective measurement of pain is difficult and all methods have their drawbacks and are essentially subjective measurements. Bishop (1959) described pain as 'what the subject says hurts' and this is after all what one attempts to alleviate in the postoperative situation.

Since the majority of patients were losing functioning lung at operation using a reduction in preoperative FEV_1 as an index of analgesia was impossible. Prolonged regular pain scoring was impractical and we therefore elected to use the well-tried linear analogue scoring (Revill *et al.* 1976) in conjunction with descriptive score.

A prospective randomized trial of patients undergoing thoracotomy has been undertaken to compare controlled-release morphine tablets (MST Continus tablets, Napp Laboratories Ltd.) with the previous standard regimen of intramuscular morphine. Informed consent was obtained from all patients who were randomized prior to surgery to receive either controlled-release morphine orally 20 mg 12-hourly or intramuscular morphine 10 mg four-hourly. Both regimens started six hours after the end of the operation and were given for 48 hours. The six-hour delay was built into the

Advances in Morphine Therapy. The 1983 International Symposium on Pain Control, edited by E. Wilkes, 1984: Royal Society of Medicine International Congress and Symposium Series No. 64, published by the Royal Society of Medicine.

protocol to allow any analgesic agents used during anaesthesia to wear off and for base-line pain control with intravenous morphine to be established. All patients underwent thoracotomy with posterior division of a rib and no patients had the costal margin divided. The majority underwent pulmonary resection or exploration but as can be seen from Table 1 there is a scattering of hiatal hernia repairs, excision of mediastinal tumours, decortications, and mitral valvotomies. Although the surgical team varied little there were several anaesthetists involved but the usual anaesthetic technique was an induction using thiopentone and suxamethonium, often with fentanyl and anaesthesia was maintained using alcuronium or pancuronium with a nitrous oxide/oxygen mixture and a low percentage of halothane or enflurane. No patients had any form of intercostal block.

Table 1

Operation	M	F
Pulmonary resection	52	9
Exploratory thoracotomy	16	2
Hiatal hernia repair	3	1
Decortication of empyema	2	0
Excision of mediastinal tumour	1	1
Mitral valvotomy		1

The patients' pain was assessed postoperatively by asking them to complete a 10 cm linear analogue assessment of the degree of their pain and also to indicate from four choices words describing the severity of their pain. The linear analogues were subsequently scored from 0 to 10 in centimetres, the descriptions were scored from 0 to 3, 0 being no pain at all.

Seventy-four men and 14 women entered the trial, the men's ages ranged from 25 to 75 years and the women's age from 40 to 66 years. Thirty-seven men received the oral preparation, their ages ranged from 30 to 75 years with a mean of 61.1 years and their weights varied from 51.7 to 95.3 kg with a mean of 70.3 kg. The other 37 men received intramuscular morphine, their ages ranged from 25 to 71 years with a mean of 58.8 years and their weights from 48.5 to 100.1 kg with a mean of 71.2 kg. Fourteen women entered the trial and eight of them received controlled-release morphine tablets, these eight women were aged between 48 and 66 years with a mean of 56.8 years and weighed between 52.9 and 79.2 kg with a mean of 64.6 kg. The other six women received intramuscular morphine, their ages ranged from 40 to 60 years with a mean of 53.8 years and they weighed between 51 and 97 kg with a mean of 70.9 kg.

The vast majority of the patients are male and the numbers of women entering the trial are too small for a separate statistical analysis. Although it was felt there might well be an inherent difference between the sexes in their perception and expression of pain this has not been borne out by the results.

Results

Analysis of the linear analogue scores and descriptive scores shows little difference between the groups receiving either oral or intramuscular morphine. There is a shift towards lower scores on the second day but this might have been expected.

The mean and median linear analogue scores show no difference within 95 per cent confidence limits and this is confirmed when the mean pain score for the oral treatment was compared using Student's *t*-test with the mean pain score for the intramuscular treatment for Days 1 and 2 separately (Table 2). Similarly comparing the median

Table 2

Linear analogue scores—means and medians

Day	Treatment	Mean (95 per cent confidence range)	Median
1	Oral	4.62(±0.68)	4.75
	i.m.	4.23(±0.81)	4.11
2	Oral	3.89(±0.72)	3.58
	i.m.	3.40(±0.66)	3.11

There were 45 patients in the oral group and 43 patients in the i.m. group.

scores using the median test and Mann–Whitney test showed no significant or near-significant difference. Using the Kolmogorov–Smirnov test to compare frequency distributions between the two groups on Days 1 and 2 again showed no difference (Figs. 1 and 2).

In no group was respiratory depression or nausea a problem. Four men receiving intramuscular morphine injections and five receiving the tablets either missed one dose in the 48 hours or had a single dose reduced. Three of these patients (two of them receiving the oral preparation) developed atrial fibrillation which compromised their cardiac output temporarily and for this reason a single dose of morphine was omitted or reduced. The other six patients refused the due dose claiming that they did not need it and they were all patients with consistently low pain scores.

Three patients who entered the trial but are not shown here were withdrawn for two reasons: one patient required ventilation and subsequently died and was obviously unable to complete the pain scores. The other two individuals' documentation is incomplete and they are therefore not included.

Conclusions

Seventy-four men and 14 women undergoing thoracotomy for a variety of operative procedures received either 20 mg of controlled-release oral morphine 12-hourly or 10 mg of intramuscular morphine four-hourly as their postoperative analgesia. There was no difference in the pain scores between the two groups, confirming the Leicester experience (Fell *et al.* 1982) that controlled-release morphine is a satisfactory postoperative analgesic. Since regular intramuscular injections can only add to the patient's discomfort we would suggest that a regimen of controlled-release oral morphine tablets is to be preferred.

The post-thoracotomy patient is able to eat and drink very soon after operation and therefore an oral analgesic is ideal for this group of patients. We have shown that the

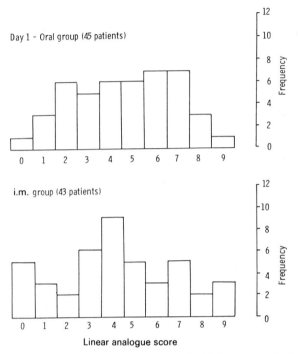

Fig. 1. Frequency distribution of pain scores using the Kolmogorov–Smirnov test, Day 1

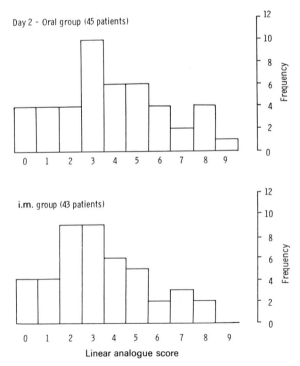

Fig. 2. Frequency distribution of pain scores using the Kolmogorov–Smirnov test, Day 2

degree of analgesia achieved between 20 mg of controlled-release morphine orally and 10 mg of intramuscular morphine four-hourly is comparable. The pain scores, although equivalent in our two groups, are not as low as one would wish and we shall continue to look for a regimen that will provide almost complete pain relief without the risk of respiratory depression or over-sedation. This ideal may be achieved with larger or more frequent doses of controlled-release oral morphine or by combining our current regimen with some form of intercostal block at the time of surgery.

Acknowledgements

This study would not have been possible without the willing assistance of my registrars and senior house officers. I am also indebted to Mr Peter Treasure of Cambridge University for the statistical analyses and to Miss Jane Blythe for secretarial assistance.

References

Bishop, G. H. (1959). In *Measurements of subjective responses* (ed. H. K. Beecher). Oxford University Press, New York.

Fell, D., Chmielewski, A., and Smith, G. (1982). Post-operative analgesia with controlled-release morphine sulphate: comparison with intramuscular morphine. *Br. med. J.* **285,** 92.

Revill, S. I., Robinson, J. O., Rosen, M., and Hogg, M. I. J. (1976). The reliability of a linear analogue for evaluating pain. *Anaesthesia* **31,** 1191.

Day-case herniorrhaphy: early postoperative pain control

P. E. M. JARRETT, C. BISHOP, and K. HITCHCOX

Kingston Hospital,
Kingston upon Thames,
Surrey

Introduction

It is most important to achieve adequate postoperative analgesia in day-case surgery. The patient returns home following this method of surgery. The analgesic regimen to be followed, therefore, must be straightforward and, ideally, only orally administered drugs should be used.

A sustained-release preparation of morphine, MST Continus tablets (Napp Laboratories Ltd.), is available. This has been shown to produce sustained plasma morphine levels (Welsh *et al.* 1983).

As a consequence of this when compared to other oral opiates less frequent doses of MST Continus tablets are required and the incidence of breakthrough pain, as plasma morphine levels fall, is reduced (Leslie *et al.* 1980).

It was felt that MST Continus tablets might be beneficial in day-case surgery. Two trials were carried out comparing the use postoperatively of two strengths of MST Continus tablets with pethidine tablets in patients undergoing day-case hernia repair under local anaesthetic.

Materials and methods

Two hundred consecutive patients undergoing hernia repair under local anaesthetic as day cases in the Surgical Day Unit at Kingston Hospital were studied. The method of surgery and the arrangements for postoperative care have been described elsewhere (Baskerville and Jarrett 1983). The patients were randomly allocated to receive postoperatively, either MST Continus tablets or pethidine tablets. The patients using MST Continus tablets took the first tablet before leaving the day unit and those using pethidine tablets took the first tablet as soon as they were at home in bed. The MST Continus tablets were taken eight-hourly for 24 hours and the pethidine tablets four-hourly for 24 hours. Thereafter the patients were told to use dextropropoxyphene and

Advances in Morphine Therapy. The 1983 International Symposium on Pain Control, edited by E. Wilkes, 1984: Royal Society of Medicine International Congress and Symposium Series No. 64, published by the Royal Society of Medicine.

paracetamol (distalgesic) four-hourly as required, though they could take the MST Continus or pethidine tablets for the two or three following nights if required or in the daytime, if told to do so by their general practitioner or district nurse.

Metoclopramide tablets (Maxolon) were also supplied as an antiemetic, to be used as required.

In the first trial MST Continus 10 mg one tablet eight-hourly was compared to pethidine tablets 100 mg four-hourly. The details of the 100 patients (50 patients in each group) who took part in this trial are shown in Table 1. The second trial compared MST Continus 30 mg one tablet eight-hourly with pethidine tablets 100 mg four-hourly. One hundred patients also were entered into this trial (50 patients in each group) and their details are shown in Table 1. Assessment was simply carried out by asking the patients whether or not the pain relief was adequate in the first 24 hours following their hernia repair. Our district nurses call routinely on the patients on the day prior to surgery, the evening of the operative day, the first postoperative day and thereafter as required. They were also questioned as to whether or not the patients had satisfactory pain relief during the first 24 hours postoperatively.

Table 1

Details of patients

	Number of patients	Age in years mean (range)	Sex	
			Male	Female
First trial				
MST Continus tablets				
10 mg	50	57.25 (26–82)	48	2
Pethidine 100 mg	50	57.71 (20–85)	47	3
Second trial				
MST Continus tablets				
30 mg	50	50.75 (23–82)	46	4
Pethidine 100 mg	50	57.12 (35–70)	45	5

Results

The results of the first trial comparing MST Continus 10 mg tablets with pethidine 100 mg tablets are shown in Tables 2 and 3. There was no significant difference in the efficacy of the pain relief with the two drugs when assessed either by the patients or the district nurses (chi-square test with Yates' correction).

The results of the second trial, comparing MST Continus tablets 30 mg with pethidine 100 mg tablets are shown in Tables 2 and 3. A higher percentage of patients found MST Continus tablets 30 mg satisfactory (84 per cent) than those who found the pethidine tablets adequate (66 per cent). This did not quite reach significance $(0.05 < P < 0.10)$ (chi-square test with Yates' correction). The district nurses reported that 90 per cent of the patients using MST Continus tablets 30 mg had satisfactory pain relief, whereas only 64 per cent of the patients using the pethidine had good pain control. This was, however, highly significant $(P = <0.01)$ (chi-square test with Yates' correction).

Table 2

Results from patients

	Number of patients	Adequate pain relief		Inadequate pain relief	
		Number of patients	% of patients	Number of patients	% of patients
First trial					
MST Continus tablets					
10 mg	50	35	70	15	30
Pethidine 100 mg	50	34	68	16	32
Second trial					
MST Continus tablets					
30 mg	50	42	84	8	16
Pethidine 100 mg	50	33	66	17	34

First trial: $p = $ NS.
Second trial: $0.05 < p < 0.10$; $p < 0.01$.

Table 3

Results from district nurses

	Number of patients	Adequate pain relief		Inadequate pain relief	
		Number of patients	% of patients	Number of patients	% of patients
First trial					
MST Continus tablets					
10 mg	50	32	64	18	36
Pethidine 100 mg	50	30	60	20	40
Second trial					
MST Continus tablets					
30 mg	50	45	90	5	10
Pethidine 100 mg	50	32	64	18	36

First trial: $p = $ NS.
Second trial: $p < 0.01$.

Discussion

From a purely analgesic point of view there would seem to be little difference between MST Continus tablets 10 mg and pethidine 100 mg. MST Continus tablets 30 mg, however, appears to be preferable to pethidine 100 mg. The district nurses reported slightly more satisfactory results with MST Continus tablets 30 mg than did the patients. The reason for this is probably due to the fact that they have experience of a large number of cases treated with a variety of analgesic regimens.

Apart from the purely analgesic benefits of MST Continus tablets 30 mg it also has other advantages, when compared to pethidine. It fits more closely the requisites of the ideal early postoperative analgesic for day surgery. This is because of its delayed onset of action (45–60 min) (personal communication) and its prolonged action (9–10 hr) (Welsh *et al.* 1983).

Many patients who are instructed to take their analgesic as soon as they are at home in bed before the onset of pain fail to do so. Instead they wait for the pain to occur before taking the first dose.

The delayed onset of action of MST Continus 30 mg allows this first postoperative dose to be given as the patient leaves the day unit. They then have time to return home and go to bed before any possible side-effects, such as drowsiness, catch up with them. The analgesic action of the MST Continus tablets 30 mg then takes effect as the action of the long-acting local anaesthetic (bupivacaine), which is used for the hernia repair, is wearing off. Early postoperative pain is thereby minimized and the patient is more confident.

The patient is instructed to take the second dose of MST Continus tablets 30 mg late in the evening of the day of operation. The prolonged action of the drug provides pain relief through the night. This has obvious advantages for the patient over the shorter-acting pethidine.

Conclusion

The present comparative trial shows that MST Continus tablets 30 mg is preferable to pethidine 100 mg for early postoperative pain control in patients undergoing day-case hernia repair under local anaesthetic.

References

Baskerville, P. A. and Jarrett, P. E. M. (1983). Day case inguinal hernia repair under local anaesthetic. *Annles R. Coll. Sur.* **65**, 224.

Leslie, S. T., Rhodes, A., and Black, E. M. (1980). Controlled release morphine sulphate tablets—a study in normal volunteers. *Br. J. clin. Pharmacol.* **9**, 531.

Welsh, J., Stuart, J. F. B., Habeshaw, T., Blackie, R., Whitehill, D., Setanoians, A., and Calman, K. C. (1983). A comparative pharmacokinetic study of morphine sulphate solution and MST Continus 30 mg tablets in conditions expected to allow steady-state drug levels. In *Methods of morphine estimation in biological fluids and the concept of free morphine* (ed. J. F. B. Stuart). Royal Society of Medicine International Congress and Symposium Series No. 58, p. 9. Royal Society of Medicine Academic Press, London.

A comparison of oral slow-release morphine sulphate with intramuscular papaveretum for analgesia following in-patient dental surgery

A. KIMBERLEY

Westminster Hospital, London

Oral slow-release morphine sulphate (MST Continus tablets, Napp Laboratories Ltd.) is a recently-launched formulation, designed to provide continuous analgesia following oral administration for up to 12 hours. While the formulation was originally used for chronic pain relief, some interest has also been shown in its use for postoperative analgesia, with variable results (Twycross 1981; Hanks *et al.* 1981).

The use of such a formulation for postoperative analgesia would appear likely to benefit from the use of a loading dose, similar to that used with intravenous infusion of opiates, since the tablets attempt to mimic the effects of such an infusion. Following a pilot study to determine the acceptability of MST in surgical patients, and which confirmed the desirability of a 'loading dose' of opiate, the present study was undertaken to compare oral slow-release morphine sulphate tablets with intramuscular papaveretum injection for the relief of pain following surgical extraction of wisdom teeth.

Trial design

One hundred and twenty-two fit patients (ASA Class I) took part in this study. They were randomly assigned to three groups. Patients were not informed which group they were to enter, but were informed that they would receive either an injection, or tablets and an injection prior to operation, and either tablets, or injections postoperatively. They were also assured that further analgesia would be available if the treatment to which they had been randomized was inadequate.

In the event, only one patient receiving MST received additional analgesia, comprising one dose of 10 mg papaveretum i.m. The three groups were as follows:

1. Premedicated with papaveretum 10 mg + hyoscine 0.2 mg im + oral slow-release morphine 20 mg one hour preoperatively. These doses were increased to papaveretum

Advances in Morphine Therapy. The 1983 International Symposium on Pain Control, edited by E. Wilkes, 1984: Royal Society of Medicine International Congress and Symposium Series No. 64, published by the Royal Society of Medicine.

15 mg hyoscine 0.3 mg and MST 30 mg for patients who weighted more than 70 kg. This group was prescribed regular MST 20 mg eight-hourly for postoperative analgesia (MST group).

2. Premedicated with papaveretum 10 mg hyoscine 0.2 mg if < 70 kg (15+0.3 if > 70 kg).
Postoperatively: 10 mg papaveretum as required (PRN group).

3. Premedicated with papaveretum 10 mg + hyoscine 0.2 mg increased to 15 mg + 0.3 mg for larger patients, as with other groups. Postoperative analgesia 10 mg papaveretum six-hourly regularly (clock group).

Anaesthesia was standardized, and included no additional, analgesics, post-operatively.

Pain levels were scored subjectively by the patient at 4 p.m. (16.00 hours), 10 p.m. (22.00 hours) and 10 a.m. (10.00 hours) and 4 p.m. (16.00 hours) on 10 cm paper visual linear analogue lines (Revill et al. 1976), presented by the researcher, or, if unavailable, the house surgeon. If sleeping, the form was marked 'S' and the patient left undisturbed. The line used was straight, horizontal, marked at the left-hand end 'no-pain' and at the right 'worst conceivable pain'. The form was explained to the patient at the preoperative visit when consent to enter the trial was obtained.

Pain scores were measured to the nearest millimetre and charted for each patient. Unsolicited comments were also noted. Care was taken to ensure that no extraneous marks appeared on the scales, and particularly that they were not folded, which would give a reference point. Very few patients experienced problems in marking the forms. One patient signed her name on the line when presented (at first presentation, 16.00 hours on day of surgery), but had no subsequent recollection of having done so!

Results

Mean pain scores with standard errors shown in brackets are given in Table 1. The scores are shown in millimetres out of 100. The oral slow-release morphine group appears to have suffered less pain than either of the other groups at 16.00 hours on both days, but this is not statistically significant. Since the distribution of pain in this study cannot be regarded as normal, medians may form a more valid basis for comparison.

Table 1

Mean pain score (standard error)

Group	Time			
	16.00	22.00	10.00	16.00
MST	6.737 (2.306)	30.919 (4.846)	21.103 (4.076)	16.962 (4.360)
PRN	10.294 (3.380)	34.706 (4.503)	20.795 (3.464)	23.087 (4.465)
Clock	10.179 (4.004)	36.724 (4.767)	20.972 (4.242)	31.320 (6.106)

Table 2 shows the median pain scores without brackets include sleeping patients, who scored zero pain, while the figures in brackets are those for patients who were awake. As with the comparison of means, the MST group appears to have been more comfortable at 16.00 hours on Day 2.

Table 2

Median pain scores including (excluding) sleeping patients

Group	Time			
	16.00	22.00	10.00	16.00
MST	0 (14.5)	28 (33)	16.15 (21)	4.5 (10)
PRN	0 (32)	28.5 (34)	12.25 (13.25)	17 (20)
Clock	0 (23)	33 (36)	13.5 (16)	22 (27)

Mean pain scores with respect to time were similar for all three groups; no statistically significant difference was found between them. A downward trend in pain scores was noted, however, in the MST group, not seen in the other two groups. Two patients receiving MST complained that they felt that the tablets were unnecessary and that they caused nausea, but this regimen was otherwise well tolerated.

Discussion

Despite the appearance of many new analgesic products on the market in recent years, opiates still provide the mainstay of acute postoperative pain control in most UK hospitals. For many patients, the provision of adequate analgesia requires frequent intramuscular injections, which are time consuming for the nursing staff and unpleasant for the patient. Alternatives to frequent intramuscular injections have been evaluated in several studies (Church 1979; Rutter et al. 1980), but the 'state-of-the-art' technique, the continuous intravenous infusion, is unpopular with nursing staff, requires an intravenous line, and is potentially hazardous.

Oral slow-release morphine sulphate (MST Continus tablets, Napp Laboratories Ltd.) clearly has potential as an alternative to intravenous infusion of opiates, by offering relatively stable blood concentrations of morphine for up to 12 hours after administration. Early trials showed us that, as with an infusion, an opiate loading dose is desirable with MST for satisfactory analgesic effect, and the loading dose which we used for the trial described took the form of a conventional opiate and anticholinergic premedication. This regimen for premedication—MST plus conventional premedication was found acceptable by patients, anaesthetists and to the oral surgeons. No significant side-effects were complained of by any of the patients in this trial, and only one patient in the MST group received additional analgesia. As has been noted, no statistical difference was found between pain scores between the three groups, comparing either means or medians.

Our conclusions from this study were that the addition of oral slow-release morphine sulphate to papaveretum and hyoscine by intramuscular injection found a satisfactory premedication, and that regular eight-hourly MST postoperatively following such premedication formed a satisfactory alternative to intramuscular papaveretum for our group of patients. The substitution of tablets for injections was greatly appreciated by some patients, while a reduction in time spent checking and administering drugs by nurses may have been achieved in the MST group.

Unwelcome injections could possibly be further reduced giving oral slow-release morphine with oral hyoscine for premedication, the necessary morphine loading dose being given intravenously immediately prior to induction of anaesthesia.

Summary

Subjective pain scores were made in 122 fit young patients following surgical removal of wisdom teeth under in-patient general anaesthesia. Patients had been randomized to receive papaveretum injection i.m. as required, regular i.m. papaveretum six-hourly, or oral slow-release morphine sulphate tablets eight-hourly for post-operative analgesia. No statistically significant difference was found between linear analogue pain scores in the three groups, and it is concluded that, as used in this trial, oral slow-release morphine sulphate may be an acceptable alternative to intramuscular papaveretum for analgesia following surgical dental extractions.

Acknowledgements

We would like to thank the oral surgeons of King's College Hospital, London, for allowing us access to their patients, and also the nursing staff of King's College Hospital for their help and comments, without which this study would not have been possible.

References

Church, J. J. (1979). Continuous narcotic infusions for relief of post-operative pain. *Br. med. J.* **i,** 977.

Hanks, G. W., Rose, N. M., Aherne, G. W., and Piall, E. M. (1981). Analgesic effects of morphine tablets. *Lancet* **i,** 732.

Revill, S. I., Robinson, J. O., Rosen, M., and Hogg, M. I. J. (1976). The reliability of a linear analogue for evaluating pain. *Anaesthesia* **31,** 1191.

Rutter, P. C., Murphy, F., and Dudley, H. A. (1980). Morphine: a controlled trial of different methods of administration for post-operative pain relief. *Br. med. J.* **i,** 12.

Twycross, R. G. (1981). Controlled release morphine tablets. *Lancet* **i,** 892.

Premedication with controlled-release morphine tablets: a double-blind comparison with dummy tablets to assess the duration of analgesia

N. H. GORDON, P. A. FILLOBOS, and J. G. MOSS

Western General Hospital,
Edinburgh

Summary

The analgesic effects of preoperatively administered controlled-release 30 mg morphine tablets and identical dummy tablets were compared in a double-blind, randomized trial involving 36 male patients undergoing inguinal hernia repair. No significant difference was found in the duration of analgesia and it is concluded that the dose of morphine used was too low due to the effects of hepatic first-pass metabolism. The potential for the use of controlled-release morphine as premedication before surgery is discussed.

Introduction

A simple and safe method of postoperative analgesia remains elusive despite clinical research. The traditional opiate regimen allows an increase in the severity of pain before each intramuscular injection and is dependent on good patient–nurse communication. Attention has been focused on how to avoid the peaks and troughs of pain by sustaining a constant opiate blood concentration (Nayman 1979; Rutter *et al.* 1980).

On-demand microprocessor-controlled intravenous delivery systems, while offering satisfactory analgesia, are too expensive for general use (Welchew 1983). Continuous infusions of opiates are effective (Church 1979) but have not been widely adopted. Fear of accelerated delivery of large amounts of opiates and problems with infusion apparatus tend to restrict their use to areas where patients are under close supervision.

Controlled-release preparations of morphine are successfully used to sustain relief of chronic pain, but the rate of absorption is too slow (Leslie *et al.* 1980) for the

Advances in Morphine Therapy. The 1983 International Symposium on Pain Control, edited by E. Wilkes, 1984: Royal Society of Medicine International Congress and Symposium Series No. 64, published by the Royal Society of Medicine.

management of acute pain. To give such a preparation postoperatively for severe pain would be unethical (Dundee 1980).

In this study controlled-release morphine (MST Continus tablets) was given preoperatively, *before* the onset of pain.

Patients and methods

The study was designed as a prospective, randomized double-blind trial lasting nine hours. Each patient received either a controlled-release morphine 30 mg tablet or an identical dummy tablet. The protocol was approved by the local Ethical Committee and all patients entering the trial gave informed consent. Patients were males, aged from 17 to 70 years, in ASA Grades I and II and undergoing the same operation, the repair of a single inguinal hernia. Approximately two hours before the operation the patient swallowed the tablet contained in the next available, serially numbered envelope. Eighteen patients were admitted to the morphine group and 18 to the dummy group. No other premedicant drugs were given. General anaesthesia was induced with thiopentone and maintained with nitrous oxide and halothane in oxygen, the patients breathing spontaneously by facemask. Patients were instructed to indicate if any postoperative pain was not tolerable. In this event, intramuscular morphine was given and the time of injection recorded. The occurrence of any side-effect was noted. The timing of premedication, the start and finish of anaesthesia, and recovery were recorded.

Results

Patients in the controlled-release morphine and dummy medication groups were of the same sex, underwent the same operation, and were broadly matched for age (Table 1).

Table 1

Patient characteristics

	Morphine group mean (SD)	Dummy group mean (SD)
Age (years)	49.1 (13.9)	57.4 (10.1)
Sex	Male	Male
Operation	Inguinal hernia	Inguinal hernia

Table 2

Recorded time intervals (minutes)

	Morphine group mean (SD)	Dummy group mean (SD)
Premedication	125.8 (27.7)	144.7 (58.1)
Anaesthesia	42.1 (12.1)	43.7 (14.2)
Recovery	18.7 (5.7)	15.1 (5.0)

No statistical differences were found between the groups in the analyses of the following parameters: the time interval between premedication and induction of anaesthesia, the duration of anaesthesia, the time for recovery from anaesthesia (Table 2), the duration of analgesia after premedication (Table 3), the number of patients who received no postoperative intramuscular morphine (Table 4) and the number of patients experiencing the only side-effects encountered, nausea or vomiting (Table 5).

Table 3

Duration of analgesia after premedication (minutes)

Morphine group mean (SD)	Dummy group mean (SD)
385.6 (157.2)	381.9 (128.5)

Table 4

Number of patients who received no postoperative intramuscular morphine

Morphine group No. (% of group)	Dummy group No. (% of group)
8 (44.4)	6 (33.3)

Table 5

Number of patients experiencing nausea or vomiting

Morphine group No. (% of group)	Dummy group No. (% of group)
3 (16.7)	1 (5.6)

Discussion

Controlled-release morphine tablets (MST continus, Napp Laboratories) achieve an acceptably even blood concentration for a 12-hour period (Leslie *et al.* 1980; Hanks *et al.* 1981). The choice of 30 mg was made early in the product's development and was conservative. It is now clear that, due to first-pass metabolism, the available morphine is only one-third to one half of that given by injection (Hanks *et al.* 1981; Fell *et al.* 1982) thus the dose used in this study is equivalent to four-hourly injections of 3–5 mg of morphine and it is not surprising that no differences were detected between the two treatment groups in the control of moderate to severe surgical pain.

Historically morphine premedication was introduced to facilitate ether anaesthesia. With potent agents such as halothane, opiate premedication has largely been replaced by oral benzodiazepines, thereby sparing the patient an injection. Opiates are frequently used intraoperatively both for balanced anaesthesia and to smooth the recovery phase. Controlled-release morphine tablets have been administered post-operatively but after a loading dose of morphine had been given during anaesthesia

(Fell *et al.* 1982). As preoperative medication, controlled-release morphine could help to sedate the anxious patient, supplement general anaesthesia, and provide prolonged postoperative analgesia. In the absence of blood morphine concentration peaks, there could be fewer unwanted side-effects.

In conclusion further study of premedication with controlled-release morphine is indicated, especially to establish the optimal dosage and we are currently undertaking this.

Acknowledgements

The authors would like to thank Napp Laboratories Ltd and their anaesthetic, surgical, and nursing colleagues for their assistance.

References

Church, J. J. (1979). Continuous narcotic infusions for relief of post-operative pain. *Br. med. J.* **i**, 949.

Dundee, J. W. (1980). Clinical evaluation of mild analgesics. *Br. J. clin. Pharmacol.* **10**, 329S.

Fell, D., Chmielewski, A. and Smith, G. (1982). Post-operative analgesia with controlled-release morphine sulphate: comparison with intramuscular morphine. *Br. med. J.* **285**, 92.

Hanks, G. W., Rose, N. M., Aherne, G. W., Pial, E. M., Fairfield, S., and Trueman, T. (1981). Controlled-release morphine tablets—a double-blind trial in dental patients. *Br. J. Anaesth.* **53**, 1259.

Leslie, S. T., Rhodes, A., and Black, F. M. (1980). Controlled-release morphine sulphate tablets—a study in normal volunteers. *Br. J. clin. Pharmacol.* **9**, 531.

Nayman, J. (1979). Measurement and control of post-operative pain. *Annals R. Coll. Surg.* **61**, 419.

Rutter, P. C., Murphy, F., and Dudley, H. A. F. (1980). Morphine: controlled trial of different methods of administration for post-operative pain relief. *Br. med. J.* **280**, 12.

Welchew, E. A. (1983). On-demand analgesia: a double-blind comparison of on-demand intravenous fentanyl and regular intramuscular morphine. *Anaesthesia* **38**, 19.

The 1983 International Symposium on Pain Control
Summary of the day

M. D. VICKERS

We are talking this afternoon about perioperative pain and we are looking at a traditional 200-year-old drug given by a different mechanism of release.

We started off with a very erudite view from Professor Jurna which I am sure—and he will appreciate this is no insult to him—if I say we could manage perioperative pain quite well with morphine if we did not understand a single word he said. The important and useful scientific information does not bear at all on the actual practicalities of relieving postoperative pain with morphine. In fact I would think that from his address MST would just stand for Mostly SpinoThylamic.

Then we came on to Professor Smith, who gave an elegant dissertation on all the reasons why pain relief in hospitals is bad, why it is terribly difficult to bring about and how there is very little hope of it ever getting better; I like to contrast him with Professor Gebershagen—although he did not come next—whose philosophy seems to be that it does not have to be bad at all. It is only a question of getting yourselves organized.

Now, this, of course, may just reflect the difference between German and British medical practice. I am not entirely familiar with the situation in Germany, but I can tell our German colleagues that in Britain the doctors have completely lost control of the running of medical treatment in hospitals. It is now nurses who teach pharmacology to nurses.

Now what has been the response to this fact is that we have to try to find some way of managing patients, knowing that we have no longer any control over the situation. There have been three responses; one is to use non-addictive drugs so that they can be given without the nurses interfering. Patient-demand systems—which means that patients do not have to rely on the nurses—and now longer-acting drugs so that the intervals of unsatisfactory treatment of episodes are reduced in frequency.

If we are going to go into oral drugs then clearly the afternoon developed appropriately because we started off by looking at the problem that might be there of the effect of oral morphine on gastric emptying, and I was interested to hear that in fact there was much more delay in gastric emptying with the intramuscular regimens.

Advances in Morphine Therapy. The 1983 International Symposium on Pain Control, edited by E. Wilkes, 1984: Royal Society of Medicine International Congress and Symposium Series No. 64, published by the Royal Society of Medicine.

I suspect that this is probably due to the fact that for the particular regimens and particularly amounts chosen, you got a higher brain level with the intramuscular route at the crucial time. Obviously, oral medication is very popular to those paediatric anaesthetists who believe in premedication, and clearly the message from Dr Hadaway's study is that the greatest drawback in his hands was too much vomitting. This was a nicely presented study and perhaps I was a little bit sharp on him—and I apologize—that he was really just giving too big a dose reflecting Dr Chayen's remark about not producing comparable drugs and comparable doses.

I was interested to see Miss Deirdre Watson managed to get away with less drugs given orally than given intramuscularly. I calculated that she was giving 40 mg orally every 24 hours, and 60 mg every 24 hours intramuscularly so I am not marginally surprised that her results were as good, but did notice she recommended the oral group principally because the nurses will give tablets while they will not give injections. We are back to the same problem—how to manage the nurses?

Mr Paul Jarrett and his herniorrhaphies demonstrated that if you give bigger doses of pain-relieving drugs you get better results than if you give smaller doses, but we still do not know for certain what is the equivalent dose of MST Continus tablets. The important thing, however, here is that MST Continus tablet seems to have a definite role because it meets one of the essential requirements of satisfying the patient.

I would suggest that if MST Continus tablets are to have a role as an oral drug in surgery, we have to know a lot more about uptake and what influences the levels on the recirculation.

Dr Adam Kimberley's dental work shows that MST Continus tablets were as good as an alternative intramuscular omnopon and regimens again meets the requirements of being satisfactory to the patients and acceptable to the nurses.

Dr Gordon's study, he has himself admitted, demonstrated that if you do not give enough you cannot tell an analgesic from a placebo.

Well, what are we looking for? One thing we need to look for first is what is the appropriate dose and how should it be given? I would opine that if we cannot regain control of medical treatment in our hospitals then MST Continus tablets have plenty of uses and plenty of interpretations. I think it has been a very stimulating afternoon.

A comparison of sustained-release morphine (MST Continus tablets 30 mg) with intramuscular morphine 10 mg in patients undergoing tonsillectomy

R. A. E. ASSAF, B. FINNEGAN, and A. HUGHES

Department of Anaesthetics,
St. Vincent's Hospital,
Dublin

Summary

The effectiveness, for premedication and subsequent postoperative analgesia, of controlled-release morphine sulphate 30 mg (MST Continus tablets 30 mg, Napp Laboratories Ltd.) and intramuscular morphine 10 mg was compared in two groups each of 16 patients undergoing tonsillectomy. Both agents provided comparable preoperative sedation both in onset and duration with little evidence of unpleasant effects. Oral morphine provided better postoperative analgesia which was of longer duration ($p < 0.05$). (This was assessed subjectively by a linear analogue method.) Plasma morphine levels were compared in eight patients in each group. These were obtained 90 minutes from the start of the study and when it was completed. This occurred either when the patient complained of pain or at six hours from the time of medication. While plasma morphine levels were comparable at 90 minutes, they were significantly greater in the MST Continus tablet group ($p < 0.001$) at the end of the study.

Introduction

The use of opiate drugs for the purpose of premedication has been part of the anaesthetic practice since the last century (Atkinson and Rushman 1982). In recent times there have been questions raised as to the routine use of such agents for this purpose (Dundee *et al.* 1970). However, morphine and its derivatives are still commonly employed preoperatively either for sedation or as part of a 'balanced technique'. This study was undertaken to assess the efficacy of an oral

Advances in Morphine Therapy. The 1983 International Symposium on Pain Control, edited by E. Wilkes, 1984: Royal Society of Medicine International Congress and Symposium Series No. 64, published by the Royal Society of Medicine.

controlled-release morphine preparation (MST Continus tablets 30 mg) compared with intramuscular morphine (i.m.) 10 mg.

Method

Thirty-two patients scheduled for tonsillectomy (ASA Class I), having given informed consent were included in this double-blind study (Table 1). Patients who had taken tranquillizers or analgesic drugs in the past month were excluded as were those with a history of atopy.

Table 1

Number, sex, age, and weight of patients included in the study

	Oral morphine + i.m. saline	Placebo + i.m. morphine
Number	16	16
Male	6	6
Female	10	10
Age	18–38	15–34
Weight (kg)	54–73	50–72
Mean	62.5	60.6

Each patient randomly received both an injection and a tablet, one of which contained an active ingredient. Sixteen patients received morphine sulphate orally (MST Continus tablets) 30 mg and an i.m. injection of 1 ml saline. The second group received i.m. morphine 10 mg and an oral placebo tablet (identical to MST Continus tablets 30 mg). The patients were screened off and monitored by the same observer (A.H.). Observations were recorded at 30, 60, and 90 minutes for the degree of drowsiness, apprehension, sickness, and respiratory and blood pressure changes. The preoperative assessment employed was that described by Dundee *et al.* (1962).

Both groups of patients received a standard anaesthetic of thiopentone 5 mg/kg, suxamethonium 1 mg/kg followed by spontaneous ventilation of nitrous oxide in oxygen with halothane 1–1.5 per cent.

The pulse, blood pressure, and ECG were monitored peri-operatively. The demand for analgesia was assessed subjectively employing a linear 10 cm analogue scale from 'no pain' (0 cm) to a 'maximally conceivable' pain (10 cm). The study was completed either at this time with the patient receiving an analgesic or at six hours from the start of the study. Blood samples for serum morphine estimations were taken from eight patients in each group. This was at 90 minutes from the start of the study and when the study was completed. Results were assessed employing the Students *t* test.

Results

The evidence of the degree of preoperative drowsiness and anxiolysis were similar in both groups (Tables 2 and 3). There were no untoward effects apart from nausea in

Table 2
Incidence of the degree of drowsiness following oral and i.m. morphine at 30, 60, and 90 minutes

Group	Minutes 30		60		90	
	Oral	i.m.	Oral	i.m.	Oral	i.m.
Marked	0	0	0	0	0	0
Moderate	0	0	7	4	6	7
Slight	7	8	9	12	10	9
Nil	9	8	0	0	0	0

Table 3
Incidence of the degree of apprehension before and following oral and i.m. morphine

Group	Preop. Oral	i.m.	Minutes 30 Oral	i.m.	60 Oral	i.m.	90 Oral	i.m.
Marked	1	0	0	0	0	0	0	0
Moderate	3	3	4	2	4	1	1	2
Slight	10	13	11	12	9	13	11	13
Nil	2	0	1	2	3	2	3	1

Table 4
Duration of analgesia to end of study following oral morphine 30 mg and i.m. morphine 10 mg, including the group in whom plasma morphine levels were estimated, and p values

Route	Duration of analgesia No.	Total	Mean	SEM	Route	No.	Total	Mean	SEM
Oral	16	85·55			Oral	9	51.55		
i.m.	16	84·25			i.m.	9	48.45		
	$p < NS$					$p < NS$			

three of the i.m. and one in the oral group. Intraoperatively one patient in the oral group required assisted ventilation during the procedure and was unduly drowsy for 30 minutes postoperatively. Postoperatively the duration of analgesia appeared longer with the oral morphine group (Table 4). However, the pain scores were significantly less in this group ($p < 0.05$). The evaluation of pain scores in the serum morphine estimation group provided yet a better analgesic effect ($p < 0.0001$) (Table 5).

As might be expected morphine levels were higher at 90 minutes following the i.m. dose. However, at the end of the study, the oral tablet provided far higher levels ($p < 0.001$) (Table 6).

Table 5

Pain scores following oral morphine 30 mg and i.m. morphine 10 mg in both groups including
the group in whom plasma morphine levels were estimated, and p values

Route	Pain scores								
	End of study				End of study				
	No.	Total	Mean	SEM	Route	No.	Total	Mean	SEM
Oral	16	63	3.94		Oral	9	34.5	3.8	
i.m.	16	79	4.96		i.m.	9	50.0	5.5	
	$p < 0.05$					$p < 0.001$			

Table 6

Plasma morphine levels at 90 minutes and at end of the study following oral morphine
30 mg and i.m. morphine 10 mg, and p values

Route	Plasma morphine (μg/ml)								
	90 min				End of study				
	No.	Total	Mean	SEM	Route	No.	Total	Mean	SEM
Oral	8	54.3	7.43		Oral	8	75.5	9.43	
i.m.	8	73.00	9.12		i.m.	9	38.5	4.28	
	$p < 0.01$					$p < 0.001$			

Discussion

This study indicates that oral morphine 30 mg provides significantly better analgesia for post tonsillectomy patients compared with that produced by the conventional i.m. morphine 10 mg as assessed by subjective linear analogue scoring. This is also supported by the higher blood levels of morphine at the end of the study (Table 6).

Oral morphine sulphate is used to provide pain relief of advanced cancer which has been advocated for this purpose (Twycross 1978). Because of the first-pass effect and the individual patient variations the potency ratio is said to be of the order of 1:2 to 1:3. This is indicated by the suggested levels of plasma morphine recommended for analgesia which range from 50 μg/ml (Bercowitz et al. 1975) to 16 ± 9 μg/ml (Dahlström et al. 1982). This lower level was achieved by Leslie et al. (1980) in healthy adults over a period of 10 hours following the administration of 20 mg controlled-release morphine sulphate. One single tablet of oral morphine 30 mg approached these lower levels. This dose would appear to provide adequate allowances for the first-pass effect and for individual variation: it is interesting to note that reasonable blood levels are achieved with the oral route which is of benefit for intraoperative analgesia. Sufficient levels must have been achieved as none in the group required greater concentrations of halothane to maintain adequate levels of anaesthesia.

There was some suggestion that the oral morphine provided more drowsiness in the recovery period. However, this was not specifically looked for. This effect might be due to the quality of analgesia allowing the patient a smoother recovery period. If this is correct oral morphine 30 mg would be helpful by avoiding a preoperative injection, intraoperative narcotics, and providing early postoperative analgesia, the latter reducing the nursing work load in a busy ENT unit.

The closeness in preoperative sedation and anxiolytic effects in this small group is perhaps underlined by a possible similarity in plasma morphine levels as reflected at the 90 minute plasma levels.

Acknowledgements

Our thanks to Napp Laboratories Ltd. who supplied MST Continus tablets and identical dummy tablets and for providing facilities for plasma morphine estimations.

References

Atkinson, R. S. and Rushman, G. B. (eds.) (1982). *Synopsis of anaesthesia*, 9th edn. Wright. Bristol.

Bercowitz, B. A., Ngai, S. H., Yang, J. C., Hamstead, J., and Spector, S. (1975). The disposition of morphine in surgical patients. *Clin. Pharmacol. Ther.* **17**, 629.

Dahlström, B., Tamsen, A., Paalzow, C., and Hartig, P. (1982). Patient controlled analgesic therapy. Part IV. Pharmacokinetics and analgesic plasma concentrations of morphine. *Clin. Pharmacol.* **7**, 266.

Dundee, J. W., Loan, W. B., and Morrison, J. D. (1970). Studies of drugs given before anaesthesia. XIX: The opiates. *Br. J. Anaesth.* **42**, 54.

——Moore, J., and Nicholl, R. M. (1962). Studies of drugs given before anaesthesia. I. A pre-operative assessment. *Br. J. Anaesth.* **34**, 458.

Leslie, S. T., Rhodes, A., and Black, F. M. (1980). Controlled release morphine sulphate tablets—a study in normal volunteers. *Br. J. Clin. Pharmacol.* **9**, 531-4.

Twycross, R. G. (1978). *Current Medical Research and Opinion* **5**, No. 7, 497-505.

Premedication by controlled-release morphine

B. KAY

Department of Anaesthesia,
University of Manchester

Introduction

Morphine sulphate BP has long been the standard narcotic agent used in perioperative pain control as well as being employed as a premedicant. It's usual route of administration for both uses is parenterally. Recently, however, Napp Laboratories Ltd. have produced (through their controlled-release technology) MST Continus tablets which incorporate morphine sulphate BP in their controlled-release formulation. This form of oral morphine provides 12-hour relief from pain. An interesting concept has evolved whereby instead of giving parenteral morphine preoperatively and postoperatively, one could give a dose of MST Continus tablets preoperatively which will provide not only preoperative sedation and, because of the long duration of action of MST Continus tablets, postoperative pain relief thereby reducing the need for postoperative parenteral analgesia.

Aims

To determine whether oral controlled-release morphine provides effective relief from apprehension when used as premedication, and whether a sustained effect reduces the requirement of other analgesic agents, and delays the onset of postoperative pain thereby reducing the need for analgesia.

Method

Fifty patients for cholecystectomy were given MST Continus tablets 30 mg or identical placebo randomly, and double blind, 2 hours before operation. Before medication control values were recorded, arterial blood pressure (BP), heart rate (HR),

Advances in Morphine Therapy. The 1983 International Symposium on Pain Control, edited by E. Wilkes, 1984: Royal Society of Medicine International Congress and Symposium Series No. 64, published by the Royal Society of Medicine.

and anxiety recorded on a 10 cm visual analogue scale (LAS). These assessments were repeated immediately before induction of anaesthesia, together with sedation scored 0 (nil) to 3 (asleep) and side-effects given in response to 'Are you entirely comfortable?'

Anaesthesia

Methohexitone 1 mg/kg, alcuronium 15 mg; additional as required; endotracheal intubation, ventilation to normocapnia with N_2O 70 per cent in O_2. Minimal halothane was used if two of the following persisted for five minutes:

1. BP increase over 20 per cent.
2. HR over 100.
3. Sweating.

Atropine 1 mg was given i.v. with neostigmine 2 mg at the end of the operation.

Assessments

1. BP and HR every minute (Dinamap).
2. Need for halothane supplement.
3. Onset of spontaneous ventilation measured from tachycardia following atropine and neostigmine.
4. Walking (protrusion of tongue on request) timed from end of nitrous oxide administration.

After operation, assessments were made hourly for four hours: HR, BP, sedation, side-effects, and pain using a 10 cm LAS. The time of administration of a postoperative analgesic was noted, and assessment stopped at this time.

Results

See Tables 1–3 and Fig. 1.

Table 1

Demographic data

Group	n	Age (years)* median + range	Weight (kg) median + range	Sex	Premedication interval (h) ± SEM
MST 30 mg	25	42 (21–61)	66 (50–75)	20 F 5 M	1.93 ± 0.1
Placebo	25	53 (21–72)	63 (52–100)	18 F 7 M	2.00 ± 0.15

* $p = < 0.05$; Mann–Whitney U test.

Table 2

Effect of premedication on anaesthesia; need for halothane supplement and recovery

| Group | n | Halothane | | Onset of breathing (min) ± SEM | Waking (min) ± SEM |
		Number of patients	Time (min) ± SEM		
MST 30 mg	25	7 (28%)	34.6 ± 8.3	0.37 ± 0.1	1.9 ± 0.52
Placebo	25	12 (48%)	27.8 ± 5.9	0.23 ± 0.09	1.54 ± 0.15

Table 3

Postoperative effect of premedication. Pain and sedation after one hour, and time to administration of analgesia

Group	n	Pain intensity* (median + range)	Sedation score†	Time to analgesic* (h) (median + range)
MST 20 mg	25	86 (30–100)	1.77 ± 0.22	1.25 (0.2–18)
Placebo	25	94.5 (50–100)	1.26 ± 0.19	1 (0.3–12)

* $p < 0.05$; Mann–Whitney U test.
† $p = < 0.05$; medians test, Yates' correction.

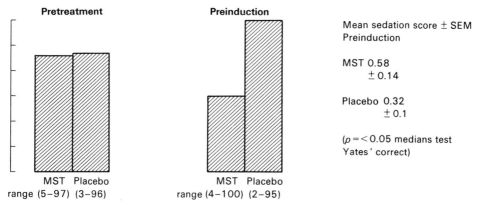

Fig. 1. Preoperative anxiety and sedation (No. of patients = 25).

Conclusions

Oral MST Continus tablets 30 mg two hours before anaesthesia:

1. Causes significant sedation.
2. Does not cause side-effects.
3. Does not affect anaesthesia or recovery.
4. Contributes towards postoperative analgesia and sedation.

Session 2: Intractable pain control

Chairmen

H. U. GEBERSHAGEN

D. VERE

The role of narcotics in intractable pain control

I. M. C. CLARKE

Pain Relief Centre,
Hope Hospital,
Salford

From earliest times narcotics have been used to control pain. Until the mid-nineteenth century these were given by inhalation, orally or rectally. Preparations were usually crude extracts of opium with little attempt or ability to control quality and thus doses were regulated in time and quantity by the clinical effect.

Over the last hundred years the usage of narcotics has changed markedly. The availability of injection as a means of administration and purer preparations has required more precision to be used to avoid overdosage—this is even more important when the spinal or epidural route is used.

Increasing drug abuse in the community has made all physicians wary of prescribing narcotics for longer than a few days and frequently inhibits their use altogether outside the acute medical or surgical situation.

In the field of chronic intractable pain the narcotics, once the mainstay of management, are often regarded as unacceptably dangerous and many programmes devised for chronic pain management include withdrawal of narcotic medication as a primary objective.

Even in terminal malignant disease opiates are still withheld until the last possible moment when they will be minimally effective. Once the decision has been made to use narcotics they are almost always given in doses which are inadequate both in size and frequency because of irrational fears of respiratory depression and addiction.

Respiratory depression is never seen when opiates are given in such a way as to just completely relieve the pain; pain itself acting as a very potent respiratory stimulant. Care should be taken, however if other methods of pain relief (such as nerve blocks) are simultaneously employed since respiratory arrest has occurred when pain no longer opposes this effect of narcotics. This should never present a risk to the patient when such physical methods of pain relief are carried out in properly organized pain clinics.

Whilst no-one would deny the potential for addiction inherent in all narcotics the enormous consumption of benzodiazepines, alcohol, and other psychoactive drugs suggests that our attitudes to narcotics may be conditioned more by fears of criminal

Advances in Morphine Therapy. The 1983 International Symposium on Pain Control, edited by E. Wilkes, 1984: Royal Society of Medicine International Congress and Symposium Series No. 64, published by the Royal Society of Medicine.

activity than by medical factors. The price of illicit heroin in Manchester is now so low that a substantial habit can now be supported by unemployment benefit and it would be more expensive to be addicted to methaqualone.

The use of narcotics to relieve the visceral pain of cancer is well established. Regrettably they are frequently misused so that patients get poor relief or too many side-effects. The drugs are then blamed for the physician's incompetence. Probably the commonest error is failure accurately to diagnose the cause of pain, so that narcotics are given for pain which would respond better to a non-steroidal anti-inflammatory drug or to a psychotropic/anticonvulsant analgesic. When opiates are correctly selected too often the specific drug employed is inappropriate for chronic pain and the method of administration ill-chosen.

Narcotics may be conveniently divided into full and partial agonists. The latter, including buprenorphine, nalbuphine, and butorphanol are often effective analgesics which may be highly suitable for acute pain or where the patient is not ambulant. The relatively high incidence of side-effects and their incompatibility with full agonists make them unsuitable for chronic malignant pain and frequently unacceptable to the patient with non-terminal illness. Whilst the dependence liability in the laboratory is much lower than for full agonists this is of little relevance in malignant disease and may be irrelevant in most chronic pain patients where the choice may lie between mobility with narcotics or total loss of all independence without. Pentazocine is a narcotic antagonist with such a poor pharmacological profile that it has no place in this field of medicine.

There are many pure agonist narcotics available but few have the full spectrum of activity ideally required. This should include high potency, low incidence of initial side-effects, no long-term adverse effects, oral or sublingual activity, and long duration of action without cumulation.

Pethidine and dextromoramide only last two hours (and the former is too toxic at analgesic doses) so neither have a place in chronic pain management. Methadone in contrast has a very long half-life (22–56 hours) compared to its analgesic effect (eight hours) and thus rapidly cumulates although some pain centres are becoming very expert in its use with the aid of blood level monitoring.

Levorphanol is effective, long lasting, and orally active but produces hallucinations in many patients.

Phenazocine is effective sublingually and may be the narcotic of choice for patients with dysphagia or where gut absorption is unreliable, particularly as it lasts 6–8 hours. Oxycodone given as a suppository is a good alternative and produces relief for 6–12 hours.

Morphine remains the standard against which other opiates must be compared. It is active by mouth, rectum, intramuscular, intravenous or spinal injection and lasts four hours (longer rectally and by the epidural route). The availability of a slow release form now gives this standard drug a 12 hour action and for chronic pain relief should now be the potent narcotic of first choice unless the oral route cannot be used.

It is well established that twice daily dosage of any drug not only enhances patient compliance but also facilitates time-contingent not pain-contingent management thus minimizing and opposing drug-seeking behaviour. Avoidance of peak and trough effects as seen with short acting drugs minimizes side-effects and breakthrough pain so that MST Continus tablets (Napp Laboratories Ltd.) must be regarded as a new preparation rather than a minor modification of an old standard.

Diamorphine is still available in the United Kingdom. For the rare occasions when parenteral use is indicated the very high solubility permits large doses with small volumes not achievable with other drugs. With oral use it is absorbed more rapidly than morphine sulphate solution and patients can tell the difference in speed of onset (whether the diamorphine is given in solution or as a tablet). In all other respects morphine behaves identically.

It should be unnecessary to emphasize the need for regular, by the clock, dosage of narcotics so that stable blood levels are obtained. Such an approach anticipates and prevents pain so that anticipatory fear and anxiety subside and may allow a reduction in narcotic dose.

Most narcotics produce nausea when first introduced but this is almost always transient. Itching may occur and usually necessitates a change of drug.

Constipation is invariable with narcotics and must be anticipated by regular prophylactic administration of aperients.

Sedation is rare after an initial period of 'catching up on sleepless nights' and indeed most side-effects associated with acute administration of opiates are uncommon in chronic users. This includes tolerance which is not usually observed when the dose of narcotic is sufficient to just abolish pain; increasing demands for drug usually indicating progression of disease. The correct dose may best be determined by allowing the patient to self-regulate their drugs just as the diabetic self-regulates his insulin. Patient-demand analgesia is well established in postoperative pain management and, on a longer time scale, is perfectly feasible with oral narcotics. Patients easily learn to control their own dose once they are clearly permitted to do so; and this has not been observed to lead to abuse.

The use of narcotic infusions via portable syringe pumps connected to intravenous or subcutaneous cannulae is effective but does not usually permit the patient any control. Epidural narcotics are increasingly used for postoperative pain although there are major hazards now coming to light. Implantable reservoirs connected to subcutaneous silastic epidural catheters present an interesting way of managing narcotic-sensitive chronic pain but again presents many technical problems. Both infusions and epidural narcotics are interesting exercises for the doctor but remove an essential aim of chronic pain therapy—that of encouraging independence in the patient.

With careful selection of drugs which are effective orally and allow the patient to self-regulate their own dose, narcotics can provide excellent control of malignant pain especially when used rationally in combination with non-steroidal anti-inflammatory drugs and psychotropic analgesics.

Narcotics can be equally effective in chronic non-malignant pain but are often withheld because of fears of addiction, tolerance, etc. When they are used they are often given in totally inadequate doses which simply give the patient a pleasant sensation (acute side-effects permitting) for a short time each day and provide an excellent stimulus to addiction. When used properly the risks are unlikely to be any greater than in patients with cancer.

If there were any alternative measures which could give the same quality of life then narcotics would not be indicated. Nevertheless there is a small group of patients with organically determined chronic pain for whom there is no alternative effective therapy. This group includes Sudek's (reflex sympathetic) dystrophy, toxic peripheral neuropathy (alcohol, diabetes, etc.), peripheral ischaemia, and the 'failed multiple laminectomy syndrome'. Most of these conditions involve a significant amount of irreversible, continuing nerve damage. All are, of themselves, non-fatal but result in such severe continuous pain and misery that life becomes worthless and suicide is a significant risk. This is non-cancer malignant disease.

Narcotics may so reduce pain in these patients that they can live a normal life, maintain employment (or regain it), and usually drive. The last point is particularly important since these patients may be prohibited unnecessarily.

It is worth emphasizing that chronic pain patients who are pain free as a result of drug therapy, irrespective of the aetiology, present as normal individuals and should not be prevented from living a normal life. There is no evidence that narcotics are more hazardous to a driver than other psychoactive drugs and may be a good deal safer than allowing a patient to drive when distracted by pain.

Modern aspects of morphine therapy

B. KOSSMANN, W. DICK, I. BOWDLER, J. KILIAN, and M. HECHT

Centre for Anaesthesiology,
Ulm University and Institute of Anaesthesiology,
Johannes Gutenberg University,
Mainz

Introduction

According to an analysis carried out by Wagner and Becker (1982) cancer accounts for 21.5 per cent of total male deaths and 19.2 per cent of total female deaths in middle-European countries. In a study of non-surgically treated tumour patients it was found that 34 per cent of those undergoing treatment were suffering from pain (Senn and Glaus 1982). Other studies have shown similar results. The incidence and intensity of pain depends on the site and extent of tumour growth. Foley (1979) has estimated that at least 60 per cent of all terminal cancer patients have pain. Applying the figures of Wagner and Becker (1982) to West Germany shows that each year between 90 and 100 000 patients suffer from pain as a result of malignant disease. Treatment forms must therefore be applicable to the large numbers of patients involved, and our main aim must be directed towards the development of methods which can easily be carried out in every clinic and by every general practitioner.

One hundred and eighty years since the isolation of morphine from opium, this alkaloid is again becoming popular in the treatment of both acute and chronic pain. It can be used in two very different procedures which both afford good long-term pain control: intrathecal/epidural morphine application, and oral morphine therapy.

The use of intrathecal morphine for the control of cancer pain, described by Wang *et al.* in 1979, initially appeared to result in a good segmental analgesia of long duration and have no unwanted side-effects. Using an animal model, Yaksh and Reddy (1981) noted that tachyphylaxis rapidly developed when daily injections were given. We have observed this phenomenon in our patients and found that it markedly limits the use of this procedure. Our patients were initially enthusiastic about the method which resulted in an analgesia of up to 84 hours duration, but were no longer so keen after the second or third injection. Only one out of 11 tumour patients was prepared to undergo a fourth intrathecal injection (Koßmann *et al.* 1982). A similarly rapid development of tachyphylaxis has been described by Ventafridda *et al.* (1979)

Advances in Morphine Therapy. The 1983 International Symposium on Pain Control, edited by E. Wilkes, 1984: Royal Society of Medicine International Congress and Symposium Series No. 64, published by the Royal Society of Medicine.

after 3-5 intrathecal injections at daily intervals. As a result of this problem, and because of the potential complications of placing an intrathecal catheter via which morphine could either be intermittently injected or infused, there are only a few reports of the long-term treatment of cancer patients with this method (Lazorthes *et al.* 1980; Onofrio 1981).

The disadvantage of having to give medication by the intrathecal route at frequent intervals led to the introduction of the epidural catheter technique of analgesia for the treatment of postoperative and chronic pain. Investigations carried out by Zenz (1981) revealed only a slight, clinically irrelevant degree of tachyphylaxis, and led to the widespread use of this method in our country. A few cases where such treatment has been carried out for up to one year have been reported. The two main advantages of this method are the long duration of analgesia and the low dose of morphine required.

We have carried out a retrospective study on cancer patients in order to evaluate, according to the mechanism causing the pain, the effectiveness of various forms of therapy (Bowdler *et al.* 1982). Pain resulting from bone and/or periosteal involvement was found to be equally well controlled with either oral or epidural morphine, the same percentage of patients in both treatment groups becoming either pain-free or markedly improving. Pain secondary to infiltration of connective tissue was also equally well controlled with either method.

We have experienced no problems in changing from epidural to oral morphine application. Patients needing $2-3 \times 5$ mg/day morphine epidurally were successfully transferred to oral morphine at a four-hourly dose of 40-60 mg. Comparable pain control was achieved in these cases when given a morphine solution on a regular oral four-hourly basis as described by Twycross (1979, 1982), as with epidural morphine.

One of the main problems that we have experienced when using oral morphine is failure to comply with the medication regimen. Our patients became acquainted with the four-hourly routine while in hospital, but the general practitioners had considerable trouble accepting the necessity of such frequent administration, because in West Germany doctors are used to prescribing twice or three times a day. In this respect slow-release preparations such as MST Continus tablets, which need only be taken twice daily, clearly have an advantage. In order to evaluate the MST formulation we have assessed whether analgesia is indeed maintained over a period of 12 hours, whether a continuous release of morphine occurs, and whether cumulation or undesirable side-effects—in particular respiratory depression—could be observed under this form of treatment.

Method

Twenty patients were prospectively randomized into either a morphine-cocktail or an MST group. Prior to beginning treatment, and at daily intervals thereafter, patients were asked, between 8 and 9 a.m., to assess their pain intensity, pain duration, and quality of sleep by means of a visual analogue scale. On the fifth, sixth, or seventh day of treatment—at least two whole days following an increase in morphine dosage—the patients were observed from 8 a.m. to 10 p.m. At 8.00, 8.30, 9.00, and 10.00 a.m. and at 1.00, 5.00, and 10.00 p.m. patients were again asked to assess their pain intensity. At the same points in time samples were taken for blood gas analysis and serum morphine estimation via an arterial cannula which had been previously inserted. Blood gas levels were immediately measured while the second sample was centrifuged, and the serum frozen and stored at $-20\,^{\circ}\mathrm{C}$. Serum morphine estimations were carried out using a radioimmunoassay method at the Institute for Forensic Medicine of Hamburg University.

Results

Patients reported a marked fall in pain intensity on the day after beginning treatment,

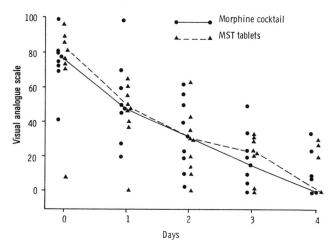

Fig. 1. Pain intensity.

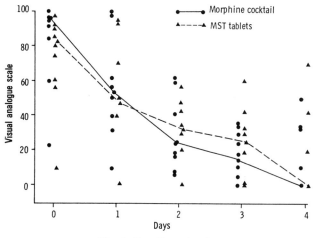

Fig. 2. Duration of pain.

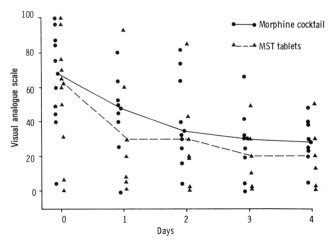

Fig. 3. Quality of sleep.

and within a few days the majority were either wholly pain free or had only slight residual pain—despite the fact that all initially complained of strong or even intolerable pain (Fig. 1).

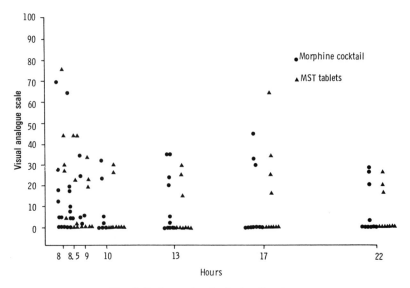

Fig. 4. Pattern of pain during the day.

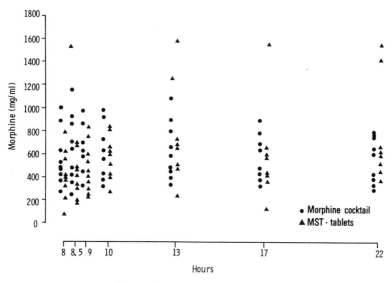

Fig. 5. Serum morphine levels.

We found a similar improvement in pain duration which in most cases was continuously present prior to treatment. The majority of patients were practically pain free on the fourth day of treatment irrespective of the form of oral morphine used.

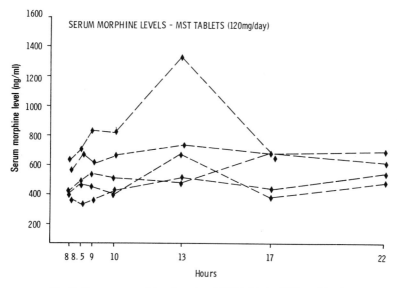

Fig. 6. Serum morphine levels—MST tablets (120 mg/day).

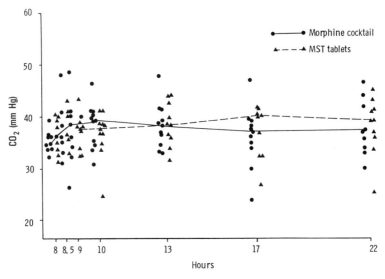

Fig. 7. Partial CO_2 pressure.

When pain was present, its duration was found to have decreased from 24 to only a few hours per day (Fig. 2).

Constant pain usually leads to a disturbance of sleep. As might be expected,

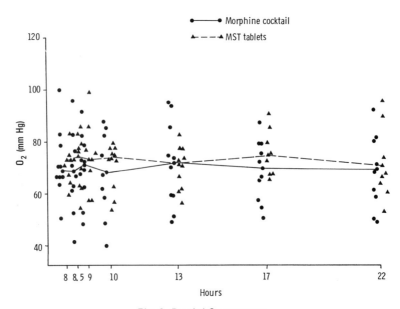

Fig. 8. Partial O_2 pressure.

therefore, we found a marked improvement when pain was controlled. Patients on MST tablets twice daily reported a more marked improvement in the quality of sleep but no significant difference could be calculated between the groups (Fig. 3).

The pain profile taken throughout the one day of repeated observations shows that most of our patients had either only slight pain or none at all. A few of the patients in both groups complained of an increase in pain at 8 a.m. and at 5 p.m. The morphine cocktail group had received their 5 p.m. dose only one hour before this afternoon pain peak, indicating that this increase may be a manifestation of the circadian rhythm—which encompasses pain experience—rather than the result of a fall in morphine activity (Fig. 4). The serum morphine levels of both groups were consistently high indicating that this is probably the case (Fig. 5).

Individual variations in morphine level are at least in part probably the result of changes in gastrointestinal motility and vascular perfusion during and following meals. Serum morphine levels and the 14-hour pain profile clearly shows that the use of slow-release morphine tablets affords adequate serum levels and a good quality of analgesia over a period of 12 hours (Fig. 6).

Serum morphine levels of up to and over 1700 ng/ml—a value never reached after a single i.v. injection of 10 mg morphine—clearly indicate that when oral morphine is taken on a regular basis bioavailability is quite adequate. Walsh *et al.* (1981) have described the pharmacokinetic changes which may occur when oral morphine is regularly taken. Enzyme inhibition may result in a decrease in glucuronization and hence a rise in free morphine levels, possibly also in an alteration in the metabolic pathway taken, with codeine being formed as a by-product. These changes are thought to contribute to the analgesic quality of morphine treatment, and can also be expected to occur when the slow-release formulation is used because similarly high serum morphine levels are then maintained as when morphine is given in solution.

Respiratory depression of such a degree as to cause abnormal blood gas levels was noted in only one patient who belonged to the morphine-cocktail group. This particular case had terminal Hodgkin's disease with a pleural effusion on one side. None of the other patients had abnormal partial pressures of oxygen or carbon dioxide such as would indicate a disturbance of respiratory function (Figs. 7 and 8).

On the basis of these results it can be said that the use of slow-release MST tablets gives an equally good analgesia and causes no additional side-effects when compared to the regular four-hourly intake of a solution of morphine hydrochloride.

Discussion

All our efforts at pain control are aimed at achieving a long-lasting analgesia with as few side-effects as possible. Two different procedures have developed as a result—the epidural and the regular oral application of opiates. Epidural analgesia affords a much longer duration of pain control per dose than is possible with the i.v., i.m., or the conventional oral route, but the development of tachyphylaxis nevertheless often makes a twice-daily application necessary. With the new slow-release formulation, MST Continus tablets, an analgesia of 12 hours duration can now be achieved. Comparison of the potential dangers and side-effects of these two different methods of treatment show the relatively small amounts of morphine necessary for epidural analgesia to be an advantage of this technique. On the other hand, using an epidural catheter entails specialized after-care and always carries the risk of infection; we therefore consider this method to be impractical. In contrast, each and every doctor is able to prescribe morphine tablets and both patients and their general practitioners find the twice daily routine acceptable.

Maghora *et al.* (1980) described the development of epidural opiate analgesia as a successful battle in the war against pain. The introduction of slow-release morphine tablets which afford a good quality analgesia of 12 hours duration must be seen as an important new weapon with which to continue the fight.

References

Bowdler, I., Koßmann, B., Dick, W., Inoka, P., and Schleinzer, W. (1982). Wirksamkeit verschiedener Therapieformen bei karzinombedingten Schmerzen. *Anaesthesit* **31,** 650.

Foley, K. M. (1979). Pain syndromes in patients with cancer. In *Advances in pain research and therapy*, Vol. 2. *Pain of advanced cancer* (ed. J. J. Bonica and V. Ventafridda), p. 59. Raven Press, New York.

Glynn, C. J. and Lloyd, J. W. (1976). The diurnal variation in perception of pain. *Proc. R. Soc.* **B 69,** 369.

Koßmann, B., Driessen, A., Mehrkens, H. H., and Dick, W. (1982). Intrathecally applied morphine for treatment of postoperative and chronic pain. In *Anaesthesiology and intensive care medicine*, Vol. 114. *Spinal opiate analgesia* (eds. T. L. Yaksh and H. Müller), p. 116. Springer-Verlag, Berlin.

Lazorthes, Y., Gouarderes, Ch., Verdie, J. C., Monsarrat, B., Bastide, R., Campan, L., Alwan, A., and Cros, J. (1980). Analgésie par injection intrathécale de morphine. Étude pharmacocinétique et application aux douleurs irréductibles. *Neuro-chirurgie* **26,** 159.

Magora, F., Olshwang, D., Eimerl, D., Shorr, J., Ketzenelson, R., Cotev, S., and Davidson, T. (1980). Observation on extradural morphine analgesia in various pain conditions. *Br. J. Anaesth.* **52,** 247.

Onofrio, B. (1981). Spinal opiate analgesia: characteristics and principles of action. *Pain* **11,** 293.

Procacci, P., Buzzelli, G., Passeri, J., Sassi, R., Voegelin, M.-R., and Zoppi, M. (1972). Studies on the cutaneous pricking pain threshold in man. Circadian and circatrigintan changes. *Res. clin. Stud. Headache* **3,** 260.

Senn, H. J., and Glaus, A. (1982). Schmerzen des Tumorkranken. *Therapiewoche* **32,** 5537.

Twycross, R. G. (1979). The Brompton cocktail. In *Advances in pain research and therapy*, Vol. 2. *Pain of advanced cancer* (eds. J. J. Bonica and V. Ventafridda), p. 291. Raven Press, New York.

—— (1982). Morphine and diamorphine in the terminally ill patient. *Acta anaesth. scand.* **74,** 128.

Ventafridda, V., Figliuzzi, M., Tamburini, M., Gori, E., Parolaro, D., and Sala, M. (1979). Clinical observation on analgesia elicited by intrathecal morphine in cancer patients. In *Advances in pain research and therapy*, Vol. 3. *Proceedings of the Second World Congress on Pain* (eds. J. J. Bonica, J. C. Liebskind, and D. Albe-Fessard). Raven Press, New York.

Wagner, G. and Becker, N. (1982). Die Krebssterblichkeit in Mitteleuropa. *Deut. Ärzteblatt.* **35,** 41.

Wang, J. K., Nauss, L. A., and Thomas, J. E. (1979). Pain relief by intrathecally applied morphine in man. *Anaesthesiology* **50,** 149.

Welsh, J., Stuart, J. F. B., Habeshaw, T., Blackie, R., Whitehill, D., Setanoians, A., and Calman, K. C. (1983). A comparative pharmacokinetic study of morphine sulphate solution and MST Continus 30 mg tablets in conditions expected to allow steady-state drug levels. In *Methods of morphine estimation in biological fluids and the concept of free morphine* (ed. J. F. B. Stuart) Royal Society of Medicine International Congress and Symposium Series No. 58. Royal Society/Academic Press.

Instability of morphine and diamorphine elixirs—the use of tablet preparations such as MST Continus tablets is considered more advantageous

T. HUNT

Addenbrooke's Hospital,
Cambridge

Elixirs are a frequently prescribed form of opiate for the relief of pain in terminal care. These elixirs may be of very varied composition, extending from simple elixirs to complex mixtures, some of which contain as many as seven additives.

It was noted that a number of patients who were discharged from hospital on specified doses of opiate were re-admitted suddenly because their pain was no longer controlled. It was thought that this was because of a change in the pathology causing the pain, or that the prescribed quantity had been taken incorrectly by the patient at home. But further enquiry revealed that there was an association between the return of the pain and the dispensing of a repeat prescription of the opiate elixir. Therefore, the actual quantity of opiate contained in elixirs dispensed outside the hospital was examined. In total 47 elixirs were analysed (see Fig. 1).

The results show that for one-third of the elixirs the opiate content was at least 15 per cent less than that prescribed.

Two possible reasons for this were considered. First, that there was a decay of the opiate between the time of initial dispensing and subsequent analysis, and second, that certain of the constituents or additives, caused early degeneration of the opiate content. These constituents included citic acid and fruit essence.

In order to prevent these problems, recommendations on the preparation of opiate elixirs were sent to pharmacists within one area health authority. This action would appear to have helped. But, because there are a number of problems associated with dispensing such elixirs, it is appropriate to consider opiate preparations in more stable form, and it is for this and a number of other reasons, the use of tablet preparations such as controlled-release morphine sulphate (MST Continus tablets, Napp Laboratories Ltd.) is considered more advantageous.

Advances in Morphine Therapy. The 1983 International Symposium on Pain Control, edited by E. Wilkes, 1984: Royal Society of Medicine International Congress and Symposium Series No. 64, published by the Royal Society of Medicine.

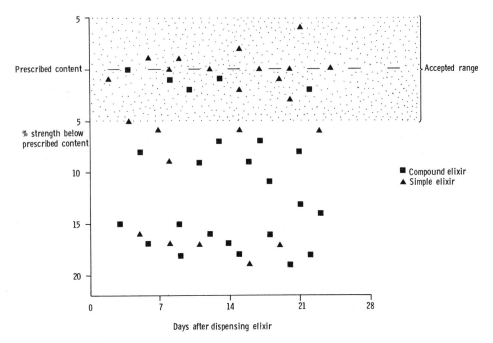

Fig. 1.

Evaluation of MST Continus tablets 60 mg and 100 mg in the treatment of pain in terminal illness—a hospice overview

R. C. LAMERTON

St. Joseph's Hospice,
London

With patients living, and dying, at home, we from St. Joseph's Hospice in East London have gradually refined the control of pain in terminal cancer (Copperman 1982; Lamerton 1975, 1979).

Five years ago we abandoned heroin in favour of a liquid morphine preparation, after it was shown that they were interchangeable in practice, because heroin is a dangerous substance to have around (Twycross 1977; Dundee *et al.* 1967). It is illegal in most countries (Tattersall 1981; Lewis 1978) and we wanted to develop a system which could be used all over the world.

But although no drug has yet been found which is an improvement on morphine, nevertheless the liquid preparation had its disadvantages. To be given four-hourly as morphine must (Twycross 1975*a*; Lipman 1980), it had to be administered in the middle of the night. And even day by day, doses were often omitted by forgetful elderly patients. So when Napp Laboratories Ltd. told us they had put our tried and trusted morphine into a twice-daily preparation, we were eager to put it to the test. At first we only had lower-dose tablets, and these proved useful. Now I want to tell you about our experience with the higher-dose tablets—60 mg and 100 mg.

Since it is ordinary morphine sulphate leeching out of the tablet, we assumed that the 24 hour dose of morphine for each patient would remain the same before and after MST was started. So every 12 hours, in MST tablet form, we would give three times as much morphine as had previously been in each dose of the patient's four-hourly medicine. This assumption never gave rise to any problems. The only time we needed to give the MST eight-hourly was when the dose of morphine a patient needed rose above what could be contained in three tablets.

Fig. 1 shows the morphine dosage we used for 630 patients in 1978–80. Clearly there was a need for some higher-dose preparations. We would like to see the development of MST 150 mg and 300 mg.

First the MST Continus tablets 60 mg. We gave these to 50 patients of both genders. Table 1 shows the range of analgesics that patients were receiving before we gave the MST Continus tablets 60 mg.

Advances in Morphine Therapy. The 1983 International Symposium on Pain Control, edited by E. Wilkes, 1984: Royal Society of Medicine International Congress and Symposium Series No. 64, published by the Royal Society of Medicine.

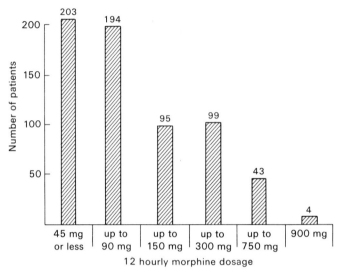

Fig. 1. Twelve hour morphine dosage.

Table 1

Range of analgesics used

Analgesic	No. of patients
MST 30 mg	15
Morphine solution	8
DF118	5
MST 10 mg	4
Heroin solution	4
Methadone	2
Diconal	2
Morphine (tablets and i.m.)	2
Distalgesic	2
Palfium	2
Narphen, proladone, temgesic, aspirin, fortagesic, and papaveretum	1 of each

Table 2

Mean morphine dosage (MST Continus 60 mg)

Number of patients	24-hourly morphine dose	Daily tablet intake
31	120	2
4	180	3
10	240	4
4	360	6
1	540	9

The mean morphine dosage during treatment with MST Continus tablets 60 mg was 88 mg every 12 hours. The values are shown in Table 2. Only six of these 60 patients were given the tablets eight-hourly.

MST Continus tablets 60 mg

The MST Continus tablets 60 mg were given for from two to 71 days (a mean of 16 days) which, for the 50 patients, means a total 812 patient-days of treatment.

Not once did a patient on a stable dosage complain that pain had returned before the next dose. This indicates that the expected bioavailability of the morphine is reliable, and therapeutic plasma levels are maintained throughout the eight- or 12-hour dosage interval.

Adverse effects were the same as those with any other narcotic drug: we encountered no special problems with MST Continus tablets (Twycross 1975*b*; Interagency Committee on New Therapies for Pain and Discomfort 1979).

When MST Continus tablets 100 mg became available we embarked upon a similar open clinical trial. Fifty-six patients aged from 15 to 82 years received the tablets. All had painful terminal neoplasia, a quarter of them with carcinomatosis from the bronchus.

Table 3

Range of analgesic before MST Continus 100 mg

Analgesic	No. of patients
MST 60 mg	21
MST 30 mg	12
MST 10 mg	5
Morphine solution	11
Heroin solution	4
Distalgesic	3
Palfium	3
Narphen	2
Methadone	2
Diconal, Proladone, DF118, Brompton mist	1 of each

In Table 3 we see the analgesia these patients were receiving before the MST Continus tablets 100 mg were started.

The mean 12-hourly dosage of morphine given in this trial was 170 mg. Only five patients needed the tablets eight-hourly, and those only because we wanted to reduce the number of tablets the patient was having to take each time (McNulty 1973).

MST Continus tablets 100 mg

Duration of treatment with MST Continus tablets 100 mg ranged from one to 240 days (a mean of 28 days). Since 56 patients entered the study, this represents a total of 1517 patient-days of treatment (Table 4).

Table 4

Mean morphine dose (MST Continus 100 mg)

Number of patients	24-hourly morphine dose	Daily tablet intake
29	200	2
3	300	3
12	400	4
11	600	6
1	1000	10

Table 5

Incidence of adverse effects on MST Continus tablets (percentages)

	60 mg tablet	100 mg tablet
Nausea and vomiting	36	21
Constipation	14	14
Drowsiness	16	23
Confusion	6	2
Anxiety	2	—
Total number of patients	50	56

Breakthrough pain did not occur. The side-effects which could be attributed to the morphine showed no escalation for the 100 mg tablet compared with the 60 mg tablet (Table 5).

For these side-effects we gave adjuvant palliative drug therapy—in no case were we obliged to stop the MST Continus tablets. The only reason any patient was withdrawn from the trial was because as death approached, some 31 per cent of them became unable to swallow tablets. Our usual practice now is to use morphine or proladone suppositories for these patients. This avoids painful injections or inhaled liquids.

We can conclude that MST Continus tablets 60 mg and 100 mg showed excellent efficacy and were well tolerated. For most patients with painful terminal cancer MST Continus tablets provide good analgesic cover for 12 hours, if an adequate dosage is used. Adverse effects were not serious—no patients needed to be withdrawn from the treatment.

But the biggest advantage, which proved to be a boon, is the 12-hour duration of action. In our Home Care Service, MST displaced all the other analgesic medications within weeks.

For patients at home a twice-daily regimen is much more reliable than any more frequent one. Non-compliance with complicated drug timetables had been a serious limitation on the service we could give. In 1980 we found 12 per cent of our patients

Table 6

Percentage of patients not taking analgesic drugs reliably

Before MST		With MST	
1979	1980	1981	1982
11	12	8	7

unreliable with drugs, accounting for most of our 8 per cent failure to control pain. By last year—1982—this was down from 12 to 7 per cent non-compliance, with consequent improvement in pain control (Table 6).

When we have a method of medication which patients do not take, physician-centred medicine blames the patients. But a more rational approach, more likely to yield benefits, is to regard the medication as a problem, and to improve it (*British Medical Journal* 1978; *Lancet* 1978). The introduction of MST Continus tablets has been just such an improvement.

Acknowledgements

I wish to thank my Registrar, Dr John Collins and my Senior House Officer, Dr Paolo Huober, for their painstaking documentation of these results.

References

British Medical Journal (1978). Pain and the dissatisfied dead. (Editorial.) *Br. med. J.* **i,** 459.

Copperman, H. (1982). Care of the dying patient at home. *Nursing Focus* **3,** 133.

Dundee, J. W., Clarke, R. S. J., and Loan, W. B. (1967). Comparative toxicity of diamorphine, morphine, and methadone. *Lancet* **ii,** 221.

Interagency Committee on New Therapies for Pain and Discomfort (1979). Report to the White House. US Public Health Service, National Institutes of Health, Bethesda, Md.

Lamerton, R. C. (1975). The work of hospices. *Oxford Med. School Gaz.* **27,** 36.

—— (1979). Cancer patients dying at home—the last 24 hours. *Practitioner* **223,** 813.

The Lancet (1978). Peace at the last? (Editorial.) *Lancet* **ii,** 698.

Lewis, J. R. (1978). Should heroin be available to treat severe pain? *J. Am. med. Ass.* **240,** 1601.

Lipman, A. G. (1980). Drug therapy in cancer pain. *Cancer Nursing* February, 39.

McNulty, B. J. (1973). Domiciliary care of the dying—some problems encountered. *Nursing Mirror*, 18 May, 29.

Tattersall, M. H. N. (1981). Pain: heroin versus morphine. *Med. J. Austr.* **i,** 492.

Twycross, R. G. (1975*a*). The use of narcotic analgesics in terminal illness. *J. med. Ethics* **1,** 10.

—— (1975*b*). Relief of terminal pain. *Br. med. J.* **iv,** 212.

—— (1977). Choice of strong analgesic in terminal cancer: diamorphine or morphine? *Pain* **3,** 93.

Morphine and endorphin in pain therapy

J. AMMON, J.-H. KARSTENS, and U. KEULERS

Department of Radiotherapy,
Medical Faculty of the Rhein-Westphalia Technical College
at Aachen

Introduction and outline of the problem

In recent years, the problem of analgesic therapy in patients with malignant tumours has been gaining in importance. The reason for this is that although modern methods of tumour therapy are frequently not able to bring about a cure, they can improve the quality of life with greater efficacy than before. This fact is illustrated by Fig. 1. If patients with microcellular bronchial carcinoma are treated only with cytotoxics, only 20 per cent will be free from a recurrence of the primary tumour two years later. If radiotherapy is also carried out, 65 per cent of patients will be free from tumours after the same period. Survival is not substantially prolonged by combined therapy, yet the quality of life is certainly improved. This is a new aspect of tumour therapy, and it should be underlined by a few figures. It can be seen from Table 1 that in Aachen and its environs 3000 out of 750 000 inhabitants fall ill each year with a malignant neoplasm. If one takes into consideration the fact that only one-third of these patients can be cured, then in Aachen and its environs a demand exists each year to improve the quality of life of 2000 patients for as long as possible.

Prerequisites for MST medication

It is vital for improving the quality of life of patients suffering from tumour pain that they can be cared for at home. Pain is controlled successfully in 97 per cent of all patients under hospital conditions, but the same is true of only half this number at home (Vere 1978). The aim of this investigation was therefore to examine the analgesic effect after oral administration of sustained-release morphine from MST Continus tablets (Napp Laboratories Ltd.). The investigation was carried out exclusively on patients with incurable tumours who were suffering from intense pain. In particular, the possibility was to be considered of releasing these patients into home care at intervals during MST medication.

Advances in Morphine Therapy. The 1983 International Symposium on Pain Control, edited by E. Wilkes, 1984: Royal Society of Medicine International Congress and Symposium Series No. 64, published by the Royal Society of Medicine.

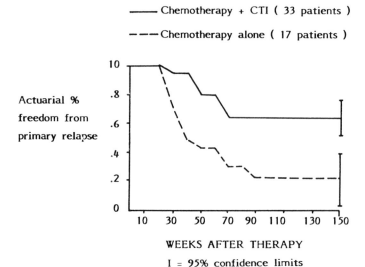

————— Chemotherapy + CTI (33 patients)

— — —Chemotherapy alone (17 patients)

Actuarial %
freedom from
primary relapse

WEEKS AFTER THERAPY

I = 95% confidence limits

Fig. 1. Percentage of patients who are free from manifestations of the primary tumour after treatment.

(From Byhardt and Cox (1983).)

Table 1

Number of patients calculated from tumour incidence who die in the course of one year in the Aachen area from the consequences of a malignant neoplasm

	Europe	Aachen area
Tumour incidence	4/1000	3000
Cures	1.4/1000	1050
Deaths	2.6/1000	1950

Monitoring of efficacy by beta-endorphin determination

In 1973, Pert and Snyder were able to prove the existence of opiate receptors in nervous tissue. This discovery suggested that opiate receptors were not created for the known herbal or synthetic products, but for a substance which is produced by the organism itself and is bound to these receptors in the course of some function or other. In actual fact, in the years that followed, six such 'endogenous opiates' were isolated from various tissues and identified (Fig. 2). These are the endorphins, which are broken down very rapidly in the body; only beta-endorphin exhibits a long biological half-life and is therefore accessible to radioimmunological detection in serum (Akil *et al.* 1979). As with opiate receptors, endorphins were only found in vertebrates. As far as we know today, the endorphins play a part in the organism's reaction to stress stimuli to which the individual is exposed in more or less threatening situations. Evidently, ACTH and beta-endorphin are released simultaneously from the hypophysis into the blood in such stressful situations. Under these conditions, endorphins are also released in the central nervous system, and these trigger a clearly measurable analgesia. This elimination of a warning system, which is essentially an aid to survival as represented by pain, actually appears to be practical in threatening situations, since in this way the individual's chances of defence are improved and his survival is assured in the wider sense (Teschemacher 1978).

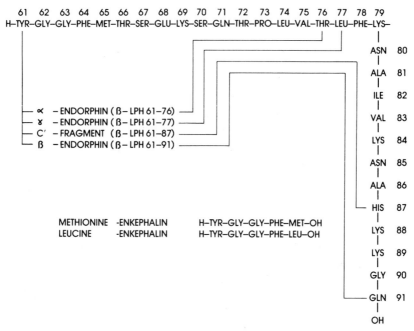

Fig. 2. *Chemical structure of the six known endorphins.*
(From Teschemacher (1978).)

In this respect, Akil *et al.* (1979) were able to show that when rats were exposed to stressful situations which they could not escape, there was a significant increase in opioid peptides in the brain. The release of endorphins can be terminated by the opiate antagonist naloxone. In man, ischaemic pain caused by a 10-minute application of a tourniquet to the arm could not be influenced by naloxone. From this and other results it was concluded that the endorphin system is not activated under the normal conditions of life and is only available as a reserve system in response to very great stress stimuli (Emrich 1978).

One could therefore imagine that in patients with intensely painful conditions, endorphins are released from endogenous stores in increased numbers. In analogy to many endocrinological feedback control systems, it could be imagined that with continuous occupation of the opiate receptors by an exogenous transmitter supply, as is the case during long-term treatment with analgesics, the release of endorphins from endogenous stores is brought to a standstill. Accordingly, pointers to an inhibition of endorphin release during long-term administration of morphine were obtained by Simantov and Snyder (1976).

Table 2 shows some well-known factors which lead to an increase in the endorphin level in blood. Apart from stressful situations, it is pregnancy which leads to the values in blood being six times higher, as do hypophyseal Cushing's syndrome and Addison's disease caused by adrenal insufficiency. Current opinion is that the release of beta-endorphin shows parallels to the release of ACTH (Hölt *et al.* 1979).

Table 2

Factors reported in the literature as leading to an increased
release of beta-endorphin which can be detected
radioimmunologically in blood

Addison's disease
Hypophyseal Cushing's syndrome
Pregnancy
Stressful situations

Table 3

Factors reported in the literature as leading
to decreased release of endorphins

Dexamethasone
Naloxone
Long-term therapy with strong analgesics

Table 3 shows factors which lead one to expect a decreased release of endorphins and therefore a decreased level in blood: administration of cortisone which blocks ACTH production, administration of opiates which, as already mentioned, occupy the endogenous opiate receptors, and the administration of naloxone. So the effect of acupuncture can probably be explained by the release of endorphins, since the analgesic effect can also be inhibited by the opiate antagonist naloxone. In a similar way, analgesia brought about by nitrous oxide can be cancelled out by naloxone. This fact also indicates that the effective analgesic components in nitrous oxide are also dependent on an increased release of endorphins (Teschemacher 1978).

To return to the objective already mentioned, it ought to be expected that patients not treated with opiates show increased levels of beta-endorphin in blood during very severe pain states, and that after administration of MST there ought to be a prolonged reduction of the endorphin levels in blood. The radioimmunological monitoring of endorphin levels in blood could therefore contribute to the assessment of MST's efficacy. In addition, attention should be paid in these investigations as to which patients can be expected to have lowered beta-endorphin levels right from the start following administration of dexamethasone because of blocked ACTH release.

Methods of investigation

The administration of MST was investigated in 22 patients. These were exclusively patients with advanced, incurable tumours. Table 4 shows that 11 patients were being treated for bronchial carcinoma, three patients for rectal carcinoma, three female patients for carcinoma of the breast, two patients for hypernephroma, two for sarcoma, and one female patient for carcinoma of the cervix. Table 5 shows the cause of the pain states. Thus in 10 patients there were osteolytic metastases in the axial skeleton which caused the patients unbearable pain. Six patients suffered from the consequences of Pancoast's syndrome in that a peripherally situated bronchial

Table 4

Basic diseases of the patients treated with MST

Basic disease	Number of patients
Bronchial carcinoma	11
Rectal carcinoma	3
Mammary carcinoma	3
Hypernephroma	2
Sarcoma	2
Carcinoma of the cervix	1
Total	22

Table 5

Causes of the pain states requiring treatment

Cause of pain	Number of patients
Skeletal metastases	10
Pancoast's syndrome	6
Other tumour invasion	6
Total	22

Table 6

MST dose required by the patients after the first week
of the investigation had elapsed

Dose of MST over 24 hours	Number of patients
2×10 mg	1
2×30 mg	17
2×40 mg	4
Total number	22

carcinoma had infiltrated the brachial plexus and had destroyed the upper ribs. Six further patients had unbearable pain because of infiltration of the primary tumour into the adjoining structures. Thus for example one patient had rectal carcinoma with large osteolytic foci in the sacrum.

Oral administration of MST was commenced with one tablet of MST-30 mg every 12 hours. Table 6 shows that after one week most of the patients were managing with this dose, and only one female patient required a lower dose, namely 2×20 mg and four patients required a higher dose, namely 2×40 mg over 24 hours. On the day before MST administration started, blood was taken from the patients during the day at three-hourly intervals for radioimmunological determination of beta-endorphin. The same procedure was used on the fifth day during MST medication for taking blood, which was centrifuged and kept in the deep freeze until the determinations of morphine and endorphin were made. The first eight days of the investigation were spent in hospital and, where necessary, the patients were called in again on the 14th and 21st day after starting MST medication. Those patients who were allowed to go home received MST for a few days up to a maximum total dose of 200 mg. The following parameters were examined during the investigation: pattern of pain intensity, duration of pain, drowsiness, quality of sleep, dizziness, and appetite. Blood pressure, pulse, and breathing rate were also monitored. Finally, any further effects were watched for, in particular constipation.

Results

It can be seen from Table 7 that 18 out of the 22 patients were able to profit from MST medication. However, seven patients denied experiencing a reduction in the duration of pain, these being the patients with osteolytic processes who said that they suffered very severe pain in moving inadvertently. Increased constipation was observed in eight and increased drowsiness in seven of the 22 patients.

The results shown in Table 8 are of particular interest. Twelve out of the 22 patients were allowed home during oral MST medication. Six patients had to continue treatment in hospital and four patients had to stop MST treatment early because of progression of the disease.

The radioimmunological determination of the beta-endorphin levels in serum did not yield any additional discoveries, as can be seen from Table 9. Both before

Table 7

Effects reported by the patients after the first
week of MST medication

	Effect affirmed	Effect denied	Total
Reduction in pain intensity	18	4	22
Reduction in duration of pain	15	7	22
Greatly increased constipation	8	14	22
Increased drowsiness	7	15	22

Table 8

Form of treatment with MST after the first week of therapy

Type of MST therapy after the first week	Number of patients
In-patient	6
Out-patient	12
Stopped	4
Total	22

Table 9

Results of the determination of beta-endorphin in serum.
The lower limit of detection is between 4 and 12 fmol/ml

Previous treatment	Beta-endorphin basal level	Beta-endorphin during MST therapy
14 patients analgesics no opiates	< 5	< 5
3 patients dexamethasone analgesics	< 5	< 5

administration of MST and during MST medication, the beta-endorphin values were around the lower limit of detection. The same applied to the patients who were receiving dexamethasone. These were patients who, because of metastasis to the brain with oedema around the tumour, received doses of more than 20 mg in 24 hours, so that complete blockade of ACTH release could be assumed.

Discussion

The results show that, in principle, the expectations concerning oral administration of MST were fulfilled. All the patients who were in some degree able to be discharged could be sent home. They were able to enjoy a reasonable quality of life in their own homes without further analgesic drugs and without parenteral administration of other opiates. Since most of the patients with advanced, recurrent tumours were given in-patient treatment at intervals, the chance of oral medication with MST was accepted gratefully by all patients. The most serious side-effects, constipation and drowsiness, were only observed in those patients who were bed-ridden owing to the severity of their disease, so that inactivity can be assumed to contribute to a more marked form of these side-effects.

The opportunity did not arise of obtaining additional information about the efficacy of MST from determinations of the level of beta-endorphin in blood. The main reason for this was the lower detection limit of the radioimmunological determination of beta-endorphin. The basal levels are to be found at about this lower limit. Normally it could have been expected that patients with increased pain would have increased beta-endorphin levels. In this case, however, it should be borne in mind that all patients, even if they had not received any opiates, had still taken other analgesics on a large scale before the blood samples were taken. It is entirely possible that other analgesics can influence the feedback control system of receptor and endorphin release just as opiates do. Moreover, some patients had received dexamethasone, and raised endorphin levels were not expected in these from the outset.

For this reason, subjective parameters will also have to be used in future in order to assess the efficacy of MST. However, MST proved to offer the majority of incurable tumour patients a further and indeed crucially important opportunity in that it guaranteed a better quality of life, even if only for a limited time. Oral administration and long-term effect are the basic requirements for home nursing, which is a decisive factor in facilitating the mental care of seriously ill tumour patients.

References

Akil, H., Watson, S. J., Barchas, J. D., and Li, C. H. (1979). β-Endorphin immunoreactivity in rat and human blood: radioimmunoassay, comparative levels and physiological alterations. *Life Sci.* **24,** 1659.

Byhardt, R. W. and Cox, J. D. (1983). Is chest radiotherapy necessary in any or all patients with small cell carcinoma of the lung? Yes. *Cancer Treat. Rep.* **67,** 209.

Emrich, H. M. (1978). Über eine mögliche Rolle von Endorphinen bei psychischen Krankheiten. *Arz.-Forsch. Drug Res.* **28,** 127.

Hölt, V., Müller, O., and Fahlbusch, R. (1979). β-Endorphin in human plasma: basal and pathologically elevated levels. *Life Sci.* **25,** 37.

Pert, C. B. and Snyder, S. H. (1973). Opiate receptor: demonstration in nervous tissue. *Science, NY* **179,** 1011–14.

Simantov, R. and Snyder, S. H. (1976). Morphine-like peptides in mammalian brain: isolation, structure elucidation and interactions with the opiate receptor. *Proc. nat. Acad. Sci. USA* **73,** 2515.

Teschemacher, H. (1978). Enorphine—die endogenen Liganden der Opiatrezeptoren. *Arz.-Forsch. Drug Res.* **28,** 1268.

Vere, D. W. (1978). Pharmacology of morphine drugs used in terminal care. *Topics in therapeutics* Vol. 4, pp. 75–82. Royal College of Physicians of London.

A controlled study of MST Continus tablets for chronic pain in advanced cancer

T. D. WALSH

St. Christopher's Hospice,
Sydenham,
London

Summary

Thirty patients suffering from chronic severe pain of malignant origin who were stable on a steady dose of oral aqueous morphine for at least 48 hours were randomized to receive either controlled-release morphine sulphate (MST Continus tablets, Napp Laboratories Ltd.) 12-hourly mg for mg or continue on the aqueous morphine. They were then 'crossed-over' twice to the alternative medication. The study period was 10 days.

It was found that when used on a mg for mg basis per 24 hours both preparations were comparable for efficacy.

Introduction

It is paradoxical that in recent months there has been pressure for the introduction or legalisation of heroin in the United States, Canada, and Australia. It seems that the substantive issue in the care of patients with advanced cancer is in fact the improvement in the methods of delivery of the drugs already available rather than necessarily introducing new or old drugs which have previously been unavailable for legal reasons. It was demonstrated recently that morphine in a controlled-release formulation could deliver sustained plasma morphine levels over a 12-hour period (Welsh *et al.* 1983). Nevertheless, plasma morphine levels are not the same thing as analgesia and there were two questions concerning the preparation. One, could the preparation deliver analgesia over a 12-hour period? Secondly, how did its analgesic efficacy, and very importantly its side-effects compare to the conventional formulation in use at that time? In Britain it has been conventional to give a four-hourly preparation of a liquid formulation of morphine, the dosage being titrated against the level of pain and the dosage individualized (Twycross and Lack 1983). The usual dose

Advances in Morphine Therapy. The 1983 International Symposium on Pain Control, edited by E. Wilkes, 1984: Royal Society of Medicine International Congress and Symposium Series No. 64, published by the Royal Society of Medicine.

range would be between 25 mg per 24 hours and up to a gram or more of morphine per 24 hours. In addition there was widespread use of adjuvant medication so it was not opiates alone being prescribed but also opiates with corticosteroids, with non-steroidal anti-inflammatory drugs as well as psychotropic agents and sedatives.

This poses many problems in terms of conducting a controlled study. One of the great problems in this field is actually that of pain measurement. In this particular population of very ill patients with advanced disease the problems are substantial, and there are great ethical, practical, and administrative problems in conducting controlled drug studies in this group. In addition to that it is important not just to measure the severity of pain, but also to direct attention to other issues such as the level of side-effects, the patient's subjective feeling of well-being, and to try and use the additional drugs which are prescribed in addition to opiates as an independent index of analgesic efficacy. In other words if a patient is getting a particular dose of morphine will that increase or decrease their requirement for other drugs such as corticosteroids or non-steroidal anti-inflammatory drugs, or indeed the necessity for measures such as nerve blocks or radiotherapy?

Method

The overall study design was, that patients who were receiving a steady dose for 48 hours of aqueous morphine for chronic severe pain in advanced cancer were then randomized to either continue on the aqueous preparation or to cross-over to controlled-release morphine sulphate tablets. Patients were then crossed-over again, thereby receiving both aqueous morphine and controlled-release morphine twice on separate occasions. Cross-over days were 1, 3, 5, and 8. The patients were followed for a total of 10 days and all the patients finished on the MST Continus formulation. This design consideration was to try and detect an effect time over the treatment period because all these patients were getting more ill as the study progressed.

At the baseline patients completed visual analogue scales assessing pain, mood, sedation, and anxiety the morning and evening prior to the randomization. The patients during the course of the study twice daily completed visual analogue scales for pain and sedation and on the intervening weekend the patients were given these analogue scales to complete themselves. During the weekdays these were completed in the presence of the nurse observer. Anxiety and mood were similarly assessed, but only on a once-daily basis. The reason for that was to keep down the number of measurements to the minimum possible because in our experience in doing drug studies before, the smaller the number of measurements you can use the better, as patients get tired out very easily.

The staff were asked for their assessment of the patient's pain, any problems with nausea and vomiting, confusion, and some assessment of bowel function. The trained nurse observer also assessed the patient's mobility, drew blood for trough plasma morphine levels, and collected the usual demographic and clinical data. On a day-to-day basis the observer continued to monitor mobility, also took blood for electrolytes, kept a constant check on the patient's morphine dosage in mg per 24 hours (irrespective of whether the patient was getting MST Continus tablets or the aqueous it was always expressed as mg of morphine per 24 hours), and monitored the adjuvant drugs which the patients were getting. The doctors who were looking after the patients had complete flexibility throughout the study to increase or lower the morphine dose, or to change any of the adjuvant drugs should they so desire. Because of ethical and humanitarian considerations, the study designed did not impose any constraints on the therapy which the patients were receiving. An independent measure was also kept of the number of diamorphine injections that the patients were receiving. Diamorphine injections were given in the event of a patient having a severe breakthrough and obviously this was another independent index of the efficacy of both the aqueous formulation and of the controlled-release formulation. If the preparation was not going to be efficacious then you would expect to see an increased number of diamorphine injections during the 12-hour treatment period with the MST.

Results

Thirty-eight patients entered the study. Eight dropped out for a variety of reasons. All the eight who dropped out were evenly distributed at the time they dropped out between the aqueous formulation and the MST. They had a very short survival after drop out and we feel the reason they were dropped was because they were dying and were withdrawn from the study for that reason. We had a final total of 30 patients, 22 female and eight male completing a total in all of 10 days on the study with complete data on all the cross-over period. The mean age was 67 years which is standard for our population and there was a reasonable spread of the number of primary sites, a total of 14 separate primary sites being involved. The morphine dose range was examined and again this included both the aqueous and the MST and was up to 375 mg at the base line, but in fact because of dosage adjustment during the course of the study the highest dose of the study was in fact 520 mg per 24 hours. There were a total of 90 crossovers, 60 going from the aqueous formulation, the four-hourly preparation, to the controlled release 12-hourly preparation, and 30 crossovers in the opposite direction.

On looking at the patient's pain assessments, mood, anxiety, and sedation scores before and after crossover, we found no difference using both parametric and non-parametric statistical analysis. The staff assessment of pain and sedation on a 0–3 scale also showed no difference in the cross-over times by using parametric and non-parametric analysis. There was also no difference in the number of diamorphine injections administered with either formulation.

Discussion

In order to design such a study a number of considerations had to be brought to bear. One is that the design of such studies should insofar as possible mimic clinical practice. There is no point in changing the clinical practice in order to conduct a study; one has to conduct the study of a controlled-release preparation comparing it to the conventionally available situation, and we opted for a cross-over study comparing the MST mg for mg per 24 hours to the four-hourly aqueous formulation. There was a balanced two way cross-over with patients changing from aqueous morphine to MST and MST back to aqueous morphine. It was randomized so that patients were randomly allocated and began either MST or aqeuous morphine. It was double-blind to patients and the nurse observer who conducted the day-to-day measurements was unaware of the medication as it was double placebo. This means that throughout the study patients were getting either a liquid which may or may not have been real morphine four-hourly, and the 12-hourly tablet which may or may not have been the MST formulation.

We relied on the staff to assess the side-effects. This was for a number of reasons. First of all because there is constant and quite good monitoring by the nursing staff 24 hours a day of the patients' pain and other subjective feelings. One important thing we asked the staff was, 'Could they distinguish between the two preparations?' They were unable to do so. It came out in fact exactly 50/50 with a substantial minority who were unable to make any comment. The number of procedures performed was so small that this factor was of no discriminatory value; in other words nerve blocks and patients undergoing radiotherapy. The pain breakthrough is very necessary in assessing whether a preparation will last 12 hours and again we found no difference in the number of pain breakthroughs whether the patients were on the aqueous formulation or the controlled-release formulation, and after crossover there was no increase in the pain breakthrough when the patient went on to the MST preparation. There was a slight tendency (these are all subjective staff assessments) to some increase in sedation after patients had been crossed-over to the controlled-release preparation.

Nausea and vomiting were not a problem with either preparation. There were only two patients that had a particular problem and that appeared to be a persistent feature right through the study and was not related to one or other formulation.

Confusion was not a problem either.

Constipation was invariable with both preparations, but not perhaps surprising.

Lastly, we kept a check on the morphine dose which the patients were receiving. We commented earlier that the physicians were allowed to adjust the morphine dosage in whatever direction they wished during the course of the study, and again you might expect if the MST formulation was not as good as the four-hourly that there would be some increase in the morphine dosage after the patients were crossed-over to the controlled-release preparation. This did not occur and again was not a problem.

So in conclusion, we have conducted a cross-over study examining the two formulations, and feel that as far as the majority of patients are concerned with chronic pain from advanced cancer, the two preparations are comparable in both efficacy and in side-effects.

References

Twycross, P. G. and Lack, S. A. (1983). *Symptom control in far advanced cancer: pain relief.* Pitman, London.

Welsh, J., Stuart, J. F. B., Habeshaw, T., Blackie, R., Whitehill, D., Setanoians, A., Milstead, R. A. V., and Calman, K. C. (1983). A comparative pharmacokinetic study of morphine sulphate solution and MST Continus tablets 30 mg in conditions expected to allow steady-state drug levels. In *Methods of morphine estimation in biological fluids and the concept of free morphine* (ed. J. F. B. Stuart). International Congress and Symposium Series No. 58, p. 9. The Royal Society of Medicine/Academic Press, London.

Controlled-release morphine tablets are effective in twice-daily dosage in chronic cancer pain

G. W. HANKS and T. TRUEMAN

Sir Michael Sobell House,
The Churchill Hospital,
Oxford

Controlled-release morphine tablets (MST Continus tablets, Napp Laboratories Ltd.) are claimed to have a 12 hour duration of action. The claim is based on pharmacokinetic data and anecdotal clinical reports. The absence of confirmatory evidence from a systematic clinical study and the necessity for such evidence has been the subject of heated debate (Walsh 1981; Clarke 1981). We have carried out a double-blind within-patient comparison of MST and aqueous morphine sulphate in patients with chronic cancer pain.

Patients and methods

Patients with pain associated with advanced cancer who had been receiving the same dose of aqueous morphine for at least seven days and who were physically able were asked to participate in the study. Those who gave their consent were randomly assigned to treatment with either MST tablets given twice a day (10 a.m. and 10 p.m.) or four-hourly aqueous morphine (6 a.m., 10 a.m., 2 p.m., 6 p.m., 10 p.m.). The total daily dose of morphine was unchanged in either case. After two days, treatment was switched to the alternative formulation and continued for a further three days. A double-placebo technique was used: all patients received tablets twice daily (active or placebo) and liquid every four hours (active or placebo) for the whole five-day trial period. Self-assessments of pain, alertness, nausea, and mood on 10 cm line visual analogue scales were completed under the supervision of an experienced nurse observer just before the 10 a.m. medication and at 4 p.m. each day. In addition an assessment of sleep was included each morning, and of appetite each afternoon. The nurse also rated the patients on a global four-point pain scale twice a day and the patient was asked to rate themselves on a similar scale. The ratings and VAS scores for Days 1 and 2 were compared with those for Days 4 and 5.

Advances in Morphine Therapy. The 1983 International Symposium on Pain Control, edited by E. Wilkes, 1984: Royal Society of Medicine International Congress and Symposium Series No. 64, published by the Royal Society of Medicine.

At the end of the five days patients who showed no clear difference between the two treatment periods were prescribed MST.

Results

The study was discontinued after 20 patients had entered. There were 10 males aged 54–80 years (mean 68 years) and 10 females aged 51–82 years (mean 68 years). Primary tumour sites were breast (five), large bowel (four), stomach (two), lung (two), anus, prostrate, uretha, tonsil, myeloma, leiomyosarcoma, and unknown. Nine patients were withdrawn before completing the five-day treatment period, but in only two instances was this during the MST phase. One patient woke in pain *before* her first dose of MST, remained uncomfortable all day and subsequently vomited. The other started vomiting on her third MST day and after a single dose of parenteral diamorphine reverted to aqueous morphine.

The results for the various assessments for the remaining 11 patients are shown in Table 1. There are clearly no differences between the two formulations: paired t tests confirm this. All 11 patients were subsequently prescribed MST and continued with it for periods ranging from five days to almost one year (median eight weeks) at doses of 2×10 mg twice daily to 2×100 mg twice daily (median 90 mg/day).

Table 1

(Mean visual analogue scale scores and global ratings (SD in parentheses)

							Global rating‡	
	Pain*	Alertness*	Nausea*	Mood†	Sleep†	Appetite†	Patient	Nurse
MST	86.0 (12.7)	71.9 (23.7)	83.5 (17.8)	11.8 (14.2)	14.7 (12.6)	23.1 (24.9)	0.7 (0.7)	0.6 (0.6)
Aqueous morphine	87.6 (8.9)	71.4 (21.1)	85.6 (16.3)	12.4 (14.0)	19.9 (18.8)	22.4 (30.4)	0.5 (0.7)	0.5 (0.7)

* 100 = no pain, fully alert, no nausea.
† 0 = not at all depressed, best possible night's sleep, normal appetite.
‡ 0 = no pain, 1 = mild, 2 = moderate, 3 = severe.

Comment

MST provided adequate analgesia when administered twice daily in all patients who completed the study. At the outset we had anticipated that patients requiring high daily doses of morphine ($\geqslant 100$ mg/day) would need MST every eight hours. In practice all but one of the 11 patients completing the study were well controlled on a twice-daily regimen. Our subsequent clinical experience supports this.

There have been suggestions that MST is more bioavailable and therefore more potent than aqueous morphine (Welsh *et al.* 1983). The evidence for this is open to question and our study does not support it. We have subsequently continued to use a 1:1 ratio when converting to MST from aqueous morphine with no problem of toxicity.

In a previous study (Hanks *et al.* 1981) we showed that MST is not suitable for the treatment of acute pain, or acute exacerbations of chronic pain because it takes up to four hours to reach peak plasma concentrations. We still believe that MST should not be used either in these circumstances or during the initial dose titration phase in patients with chronic cancer pain. However, once patients are on a stable dose of narcotic, MST given twice a day provides a suitable alternative to four-hourly aqueous morphine or diamorphine.

References

Clarke, I. M. C. (1981). Slow-release morphine. *Br. med. J.* **283,** 1549.

Hanks, G. W., Rose, N. M., Aherne, G. W., Piall, E. M., Fairfield, S., and Trueman, T. (1981). Controlled release morphine tablets: a double blind trial in dental surgery patients. *Br. J. Anaesth.* **53,** 1259.

Walsh, T. D. (1981). Slow-release morphine. *Br. med. J.* **283,** 1187.

Welsh, J., Stuart, J. F. B., Habeshaw, T., Blackie, R., Whitehill, D., Setanoians, A., Milsted, R. A. V., and Calman, K. C. (1983). A comparative pharmacokinetic study of morphine sulphate solution and MST Continus 30 mg tablets in conditions expected to allow steady-state drug levels. Royal Society of Medicine International Congress and Symposium Series No. 58, p. 9. Royal Society of Medicine/Academic Press, London.

The relief of pain by subcutaneous infusion of diamorphine

R. J. DICKSON, B. HOWARD, and J. CAMPBELL

*Mount Vernon Hospital,
Northwood,
Middlesex*

From time to time in the management of chronic pain in terminal malignant disease one encounters patients who require parenteral medication. Beside the inconvenience and time-consuming burden on the nursing staff that this imposes, these patients are frequently dehydrated and wasted with little subcutaneous soft tissue and repeated injections can be most uncomfortable. The alternative method of administration of opiate suppositories is frequently satisfactory in achieving pain control but although nurses are accustomed to rectal insertions, relatives frequently find such procedure obnoxious. We should like to report our experience with continuous subcutaneous infusion of narcotics at Michael Sobell House, Mount Vernon Hospital, a purpose-built unit for the care of patients with advanced and incurable disease.

In 1979, Dr Martin Wright described his design of a battery-operated syringe-driver, for use in treating thalassaemia with infusions of desferrioxamine (Wright and Callan 1979). Our colleague Dr P. S. B. Russell (1979) first realized that this pump could be used for continuous narcotic administration, and since that time the same apparatus has found many uses—for heparin infusions, insulin injections, cancer chemotherapy, and postoperative analgesia (Davenport and Wright 1979) amongst others.

The whole apparatus, including a PP3 alkaline battery, weighs only 175 g. The battery operates a plunger which delivers pulsed doses of about 0.01 ml of the contents of the syringe, the speed of travel being readily adjustable between 1 and 99 mm in one hour. In our practice a travel of 2 mm/h onward progress is chosen; a 10 ml syringe barrel measures 50 mm and thus the contents at this setting are delivered in 25 hours. A holster is provided so that the apparatus can be carried inconspicuously.

This method has several benefits:

1. It obviates repeated injections.

2. It is readily portable so that the patient can remain ambulant if otherwise sufficiently well.

3. The site of injection has to be changed only infrequently, often only every three weeks.

Advances in Morphine Therapy. The 1983 International Symposium on Pain Control, edited by E. Wilkes, 1984: Royal Society of Medicine International Congress and Symposium Series No. 64, published by the Royal Society of Medicine.

4. A 24-hour dose can be given and the syringe be replaced only once daily.

5. A visual signal confirms that the apparatus is operative, and in the latest model an audible alarm signifies that it is malfunctioning.

6. The speed of delivery can be readily adjusted. The driving rate is calculated by dividing the required length of travel of the piston by the time of delivery in hours. Different sizes of syringe can therefore be used over variable periods of time.

7. The blood level of narcotic remains at a constant level, avoiding the peaks and troughs of intermittent injections.

Indications for use

These can be summarized as:
1. Inability of patient to swallow oral medication because of:
   (a) obstruction;
   (b) persistent vomiting;
   (c) mouth and throat lesions;
   (d) coma.
2. Unsatisfactory response to oral dosage.
3. Terminal illness.

Additives

In our experience the continuous infusion of narcotics reduces the incidence of nausea expected from the exhibition of opiates. This is presumably because of the avoidance of sudden changes in blood level, for it is common experience that a tolerance to the emetic side-effects of opiates is readily acquired and if the level in the blood remains relatively constant this tolerance develops more quickly. For this reason the addition of antiemetics is rarely necessary. If the patient does complain of nausea we use an injection of prochlorperazine or metaclopramide given separately from the syringe-driver. This is done because there is considerable evidence that the admixture of antiemetics to opiate so alters the pH of the solution as to cause precipitation and blockage of the cannula, or irritation, thus requiring more frequent re-siting (Hutchinson *et al.* 1981; Dickson and Russell 1982).

Narcotic of choice

Because of its ready solubility, our experience has been gained almost exclusively with diamorphine. In severe pain when doses of over 1 g/day are required, this can be dissolved in 10 ml of water whereas the maximum solubility of morphine sulphate is 300 mg in 10 ml and if a larger dose is required either a larger syringe must be used or the time of administration be shortened. However, there seems to be no theoretical reason why other opiate narcotics cannot be used. The comparatively short half-life of pethidine which makes this drug so unsuitable for the control of chronic pain is no bar and it has been used successfully in the syringe pump postoperatively (Davenport and Wright 1979).

Technique

Most patients will have been receiving narcotics orally before the necessity of parenteral administration becomes apparent. Many will have been submitted to injections also. The dosage of narcotic is calculated as equivalent to that required by injection or 75 per cent of the oral dose. One loading four-hourly dose is then given subcutaneously to raise the plasma level rapidly. The driving rate of the pump is then calculated and the decade switches set at the correct speed. After the syringe is charged with the required dose the cannula is connected and filled and the butterfly needle inserted subcutaneously into the abdominal or anterior chest wall and the syringe strapped to the pump. The motor is then started and checked, the apparatus placed in the plastic case and into the shoulder holster. A fresh syringe is loaded similarly after the expiry of the time and the dosage of narcotic can then be adjusted upwards or downwards to conform with the patient's symptoms.

Experiences

Since the first patient was treated in August 1978 the syringe driver has been used for approximately 100 patients. Of these nearly half were treated in other wards in Mount Vernon Hospital and other local hospitals and by general practitioners in the patient's home, admission to hospital never becoming necessary. This confirms the great value for the patient of this method of pain control, allowing him to remain in his home, often fully ambulant.

Full records are not available for these patients but the notes of those treated in Michael Sobell House have been carefully studied and the following conclusions drawn:

1. Pain control was achieved in nearly all cases.

2. Variation in dosage of diamorphine was necessary, either upwards or downwards, in most instances but in some pain control was achieved until death by daily administration of the initial dose.

3. If other methods of pain relief were used—radiotherapy to bony metastases, nerve block, etc. reduction of dosage was achieved without any evidence of withdrawal symptoms.

4. The most frequent indication for the use of the syringe driver was the inadequate response of bony pain to oral medication and this type of pain was most successfully relieved by subcutaneous infusion.

5. The most intractable pain was that due to massive pelvic disease, chiefly from gynaecological causes.

6. Dosage varied from 30 mg to 6 grams daily of diamorphine.

7. Duration of treatment varied from 24 hours to five months.

8. Site blockage was seldom a problem although evidence of an allergic response to the butterfly needle was evident in one patient.

9. The electronic system of the apparatus has not in our experience ever failed: occasional interruption of the narcotic supply was always due to blockage of the needle, disconnection of the cannula by a confused patient, or, most commonly to the battery being inadequately charged and requiring replacement.

The success of the device can be exemplified by two patients, the first a 30-year-old female with advanced carcinoma of the cervix who was enabled to join her family on holiday in a caravan only 10 days before she died. Secondly, an elderly gentleman with obstructing carcinoma of the oesophagus who was a keen gardener. He remained at home, pain free, attended a garden show on a Saturday, worked in his own garden on the Sunday and died on Monday.

Success was not however universal. A 45-year-old female radiographer diagnosed her own oesophageal carcinoma which was treated by surgical excision but she developed widespread bony metastases five months later. The pain from these lesions was controlled by local radiotherapy initially but she was admitted to Michael Sobell House in severe left-sided chest pain inadequately relieved by 60 mg of diamorphine four-hourly orally. The oral dosage was increased to 270 mg four-hourly without relief and the syringe pump was then started, 1500 mg being given every 24 hours. Even when this was increased to 6 g daily she remained in pain but remarkably, even on this very high dosage she remained conscious, her respiration rate was unaffected, and her pupils remained dilated. Intravenous dosage of 1200 mg every four hours provided no improvement and it was necessary to sedate her with intravenous diazepam 10 mg every four hours to ensure her comfort. At autopsy the cause of her pain was demonstrated to be direct involvement of the intercostal nerves from a mass of recurrent tumour adjacent to the vertebral column, but the reason for the lack of physiological response to such a massive narcotic dosage remains obscure.

In conclusion, we feel that this method of pain control is a significant improvement over repeated injections, or the use of suppositories which many find undignified, and that it often enables the patient to remain at home in comfort. Its use in those few whose pain cannot be controlled by oral medication can therefore be strongly recommended particularly in domiciliary care. Much still remains to be learned, however. Alternatives to diamorphine should be investigated, the problems of admixture of other drugs with the narcotic need to be clarified, and, in particular, the pharmacokinetics of morphine and its derivatives require much more study than has hitherto been given. For instance, is absorption affected by the diluent of the injection: sterile water, normal saline or 5 per cent glucose as advocated in a recent report (Campbell et al. 1983)? Because morphine has been effectively used for so many years for pain relief there has been remarkably little study of its mode of action. This is being rectified and it is to be hoped further investigations now under way will lead to a better understanding of the optimum methods of using this method of pain control.

Acknowledgements

We should like to thank Dr P. S. B. Russell for revising this short report, and also Miss Audrey Day, Chief Pharmacist at Mount Vernon Hospital for her interest and encouragement.

References

Campbell, C. F., Mason, J. B., and Weiler, J. M. (1983). Continuous subcutaneous infusion of morphine for the pain of terminal malignancy. *Annls intern. Med.* **98,** 51.

Davenport, H. T. and Wright, B. M. (1979). Relief of postoperative pain. *Br. med. J.* **i,** 1561.

Dickson, R. J. and Russell P. S. B. (1982). Continuous subcutaneous analgesics for terminal care at home. *Lancet* **i,** 165.

Hutchinson, H. T., Leedham, G. D. and Knight, A. M. (1979). Continuous subcutaneous analgesics and antiemetics in domiciliary terminal care. *Lancet* **ii,** 1279.

Russell, P. S. B. (1979). Analgesia in terminal malignant disease. *Br. med. J.* **i,** 1561.

Wright, B. M. and Callan, K. (1979). Slow drug infusion using a portable syringe driver. *Br. med. J.* **ii,** 582.

Extrahepatic morphine metabolism?

**H. J. McQUAY,*† R. A. MOORE,*† R. E. S. BULLINGHAM,*†
J. W. SEAR,† and H. W. SYMONDS‡**

**Oxford Regional Pain Relief Unit,
Abingdon Hospital,
Abingdon, Oxford*

*†Nuffield Departments of Clinical Biochemistry and Anaesthetics,
Radcliffe Infirmary,
Oxford*

*‡Agricultural Research Council,
Institute for Research on Animal Diseases,
Compton,
Newbury,
Berkshire.*

Summary

Two studies suggesting that the role of the kidney may be more important in the metabolism of morphine at therapeutic plasma morphine concentrations were presented.

In the chronically cannulated cow, the hepatic extraction ratio for intravenous boluses of morphine and four other narcotics fell as portal vein drug concentration decreased. An extraction ratio close to zero for morphine was observed at a portal vein plasma morphine concentration of about 200 nmol/l, within the range for therapeutic effect.

Plasma morphine concentrations after intravenous administration were measured in patients undergoing renal transplantation and in controls. In both transplant patients and controls plasma morphine fell in the first 10 minutes after injection, but in the transplant patients there was then no significant further fall until between three and five hours. There was then an abrupt reversion to the same elmination half-life as the controls, coinciding with the recovery of renal function following the period of cold ischaemia. In the transplant patients the 24-hour AUC was significantly higher and plasma clearance significantly lower than in controls.

Advances in Morphine Therapy. The 1983 International Symposium on Pain Control, edited by E. Wilkes, 1984: Royal Society of Medicine International Congress and Symposium Series No. 64, published by the Royal Society of Medicine.

Introduction

Morphine metabolism in man is by conjugation to morphine glucuronide. This is widely assumed to be an exclusively hepatic process, with the glucuronide being excreted in the urine; the implication is that hepatic dysfunction but not renal dysfunction should lead to delay in metabolism with sequelae of extended narcotic effect.

This paper presents recent evidence obtained from studies in patients and in chronically cannulated cows which suggests that the liver may be less and the kidney more important in morphine metabolism at therapeutic plasma morphine concentrations than previously acknowledged.

Opioid hepatic extraction ratio in the chronically cannulated cow

Methods

Two adult non-lactating cows (Cow A, Friesian × Ayrshire, weight 586 kg; Cow B Ayrshire, weight 445 kg) were used. The carotid artery, jugular, hepatic, and portal (at porta hepatis) veins were cannulated in both cows. In Cow B the mesenteric vein was also cannulated. The cannulation method used was a combination of previously published methods (Symonds and Baird 1973; Baird *et al.* 1975). The animals were allowed to recover from surgery for at least three weeks and to return to normal feeding before the studies began.

Experiment 1

Cow A was given intravenous (i.v.) bolus doses of narcotics. Each dose (scaled up on weight basis to approximate a normal human parenteral dose) was given at least one week apart. The dose was given intravenously over one minute into the non-cannulated jugular vein in a volume of 20 ml, dilute with 0.9 per cent w/v saline. Blood samples were taken simultaneously from the catheters in the portal and hepatic veins. The sampling times were 1, 2, 3, 5, 7.5, 10, 15, 20, 30, 40, 60, 90, 120, 150, and 180 minutes from the end of the injection. Samples were taken into lithium heparin tubes, and kept on ice for 2–4 hours until centrifugation; the plasma was then stored at $-20\,^{\circ}\mathrm{C}$ until assay.

The drugs given were: morphine sulphate pentahydrate 100 mg (264 micromoles, Evans Medical, Greenford), diamorphine hydrochloride monohydrate 50 mg (120 micromoles, Evans Medical, Greenford), methadone hydrochloride 50 mg (145 micromoles, Physeptone, Wellcome Medical Division, Crewe), fentanyl 1 mg as base (3 micromoles, Sublimaze, Janssen Pharmaceutical, Marlow), buprenorphine hydrochloride 3 mg as base (6 micromoles, Temgesic, Reckitt & Colman Pharmaceutical Division, Hull).

Experiment 2

Cow B was given a series of i.v. bolus or infusion doses of morphine sulphate pentahydrate, and there was an interval of at least three days between study days. The study days were:

1. 75 mg i.v. bolus.
2. Infusion study (I).

3. 75 mg i.v. bolus.
4. Infusion studies (II and III) preceded by 75 mg i.v. bolus.
5. 150 mg i.v. bolus.
6. 150 mg i.v. bolus.

Bolus doses were given as above. Sampling, sampling times and the treatment of samples were as for Experiment 1. Infusion studies were performed using an infusion into the mesenteric vein from a calibrated Harvard pump fitted with glass syringes. Blood samples were taken from the catheters in the portal and hepatic veins.

Infusion study I used 50 mg morphine sulphate pentahydrate in 500 ml 0.9 percent saline solution (264 nmol morphine/ml). Eight increasing infusion rates between 0.19 and 38 ml/min (50.2–10032 nmol/min) were used. Infusion study II and infusion study III were performed on the same day, and followed three hours after a bolus i.v. injection of 75 mg of morphine sulphate. Infusion study II used 30 mg morphine sulphate in 500 ml 0.9 per cent saline solution (158 nmol morphine/ml). The infusion rates used were 9.6, 19.1, and 38 ml/min (1517, 3018, and 6004 nmol/min). Infusion study III used 60 mg morphine sulphate in 500 ml 0.9 per cent saline solution (317 nmol morphine/ml). Five increasing infusion rates of 1.9–38 ml/min (602–12046 nmol/min) were used. In each study samples were taken approximately five and ten minutes after infusion rate change. In addition, syringe pumps were used to withdraw blood at constant flow rate from the portal and hepatic lines for five minutes between the five and ten minute sample times. The samples were treated as in Experiment 1.

Portal and hepatic blood flows were estimated in Cow B during the first 75 mg i.v. bolus study by the dilution of para-aminohippurate infused into the mesenteric vein. The samples were taken at the same times as those for morphine estimation, and were treated in the same way.

Assays

All the plasma opiate concentrations were determined by radioimmunoassay using the methods cited: buprenorphine (Bartlett *et al.* 1980), fentanyl (McQuay *et al.* 1979), methadone (Bullingham *et al.* 1982), and morphine (Moore *et al.* 1984*a*). Diamorphine was measured as morphine equivalents; the cross-reactivity was 100 per cent in this morphine assay. For all methods the inter- and intra-assay coefficients of variation were less than 10 per cent at several drug concentrations.

For each simultaneous portal and hepatic vein sample pair, the extraction ratio was calculated as:

$$\text{Hepatic extraction ratio (HER)} = (C_p - C_h)/C_p$$

where C_p and C_h were the opioid drug concentrations in portal and hepatic veins.

Results

In Experiment 1 the tendency for all five drugs was for lower HER with lower portal plasma drug concentration (Fig. 1). Experiment 2 showed the same relationship for morphine when different drug delivery sequences were used (Fig. 2).

HER values at or close to zero were obtained at the lowest observed concentrations, except for methadone. Graphical extrapolation produced a concentration (C_{pass}) at which HER was predicted to be zero. Similarly a maximum HER value (HER_{max}) was observed (Table 1). Separate values are given for the bolus and infusion results for Experiment 2.

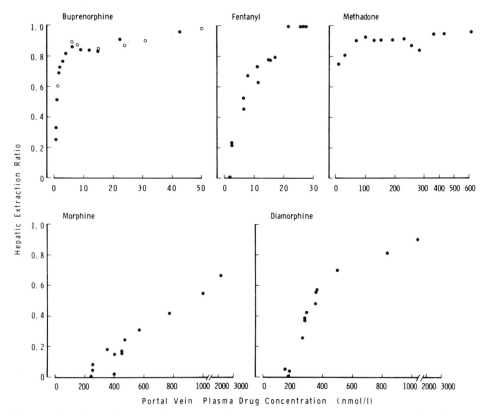

Fig. 1. Transhepatic extraction ratios for five narcotics in the cow calculated from simultaneous portal and hepatic vein drug concentrations. For buprenorphine open and closed circles represent two separate experiments.

The mean values of the 10 separate estimates of hepatic and portal venous blood flow were 15.8 ± 1.9 and 12.4 ± 2.2 (sd, 1/min) respectively; there was no systematic relation to either measurement time or plasma morphine concentration.

Conclusions

These studies demonstrate concentration dependent transhepatic extraction for five narcotics in the cow *in vivo*, HER decreasing as portal vein plasma drug concentration falls.

The finding of HER concentration dependence with five different narcotics shows that the phenomenon was not specific to one drug, but could still be specific to narcotics. The reproduction of the phenomenon in more than one cow shows that it was not an artefact of the model in one cow. The measurement of hepatic blood flow from the same vessel lines as used for drug sampling showed that at 14 1/min the flow was in the normal range for the cow; the concentration dependence of HER could not therefore be attributed to an aberration in the citing of the sampling catheters. While the drug measurements were all radioimmunoassays, the fact that all the assays were different with no common factor such as a standard extraction regimen means that the

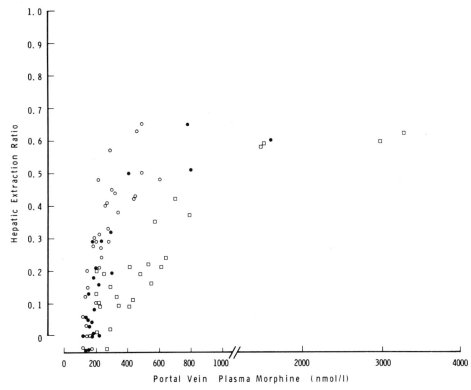

Fig. 2. Transhepatic extraction ratios for morphine calculated from simultaneous portal and hepatic vein drug concentrations. Symbols indicate results from bolus doses (o, ●) and increasing infusions (□).

Table 1

Estimated plasma values for C_{pass} and HER_{max}

	C_{pass} (nmol/l)	HER_{max}
Experiment 1		
Buprenorphine	0.4	0.9
Methadone	0.9	0.9
Fentanyl	2.1	1.0
Diamorphine	190	0.8
Morphine	210	0.6
Experiment 2		
75 mg i.v. bolus	150	0.7
75 mg i.v. bolus	180	0.6
150 mg i.v. bolus	170	0.6
150 mg i.v. bolus	170	0.6
Infusion studies		
I	170	0.65
II	170	0.6
III	180	0.5

phenomenon is unlikely to be an assay artefact. The finding (Fig. 2) of essentially the same C_{pass} and HER_{max} values for morphine in infusion with ascending concentrations, with and without i.v. bolus preload, as were seen in i.v. bolus studies alone showed that the phenomenon was not restricted to descending drug concentrations after bolus doses.

The finding of high oral relative bioavailability for morphine in man (Sawe et al. 1981; and see below) can be explained by this phenomenon of lower HER as the portal vein concentration falls, because at plasma morphine concentrations below C_{pass} minimal hepatic metabolism would occur. At low oral morphine dosage the prediction is that oral bioavailability would be maximal. The pharmacodynamic evidence supports this contention; oral/parenteral equivalences based on the assumption of fixed extraction ratios are not valid clinically for morphine. The oral dosage required tends to be considerably lower than expected from parenteral requirements and an estimate of 0.7 for the morphine HER (Stanski et al. 1976). The confusion may arise because classic analgesic methodology in a six-hour single-dose comparison of intramuscular and oral morphine would underestimate analgesia from the oral dose, which may not achieve peak plasma morphine concentration until the study is nearly half over, but which will continue to be effective, and perhaps more so than the i.m. dose, after the end of the study period.

Morphine kinetics during and after renal transplantation

The hypothesis that the liver does not metabolize morphine at low plasma morphine concentrations (below C_{pass}) and that the kidney might then be the prime site for morphine metabolism could be tested in patients undergoing renal transplantation. They have normal hepatic function but are anuric until the transplanted kidney begins to work. The prediction would be of failure to clear morphine until renal function is restored.

Patients and methods

Transplant patients

Fifteen patients (nine male, six female) gave informed consent to participate in this study, which was approved by the local ethics committee. All were suffering from end-stage renal failure and receiving treatment by either haemodialysis or continuous ambulatory peritoneal dialysis; they were dialysed within 12 hours of induction of anesthesia. Demographic data, and the preoperative haemoglobin, urea and creatinine values, together with any intercurrent medication are shown in Table 2.

Premedication was with diazepam 10 mg orally two hours before surgery. Anaesthesia was induced with thiopentone and muscle relaxant, and maintained with 60 per cent nitrous oxide in oxygen supplemented with halothane 0.5 per cent as required using the Bain circuit. The operation of renal transplantation was carried out through a loin incision and the donor kidney anastamosed to the iliac vessels extraperitoneally.

A single dose of morphine sulphate pentahydrate BP (Evans Medical, Greenford, Middlesex) was diluted to 10 ml with normal saline and injected into a flowing peripheral infusion over a period of 20 seconds. Six patients received 10 mg and the remaining nine 20 mg. Central venous samples (1 ml) were collected into tubes containing lithium heparin anticoagulant and the samples separated by centrifugation;

Table 2

Demographic parameters for transplant patients

Patient	Dose (mg)	Age (years)	Sex	L/C	Urea (mmol/l)	Creatinine (μmol/l)	Haemoglobin (g/dl)
PF	10	47	M	C	16.6	544	5.5
GG	10	51	F	C	17.1	526	6.9
EW	10	34	M	C	16.0	730	7.3*
SR	10	29	M	C	26.1	1359	7.6
SD	10	52	F	C	12.0	652	6.7
PC	10	19	M	L	18.2	1020	8.2†
CW	20	42	F	C	10.9	380	7.8†
MC	20	35	F	L	23.7	641	8.1
IH	20	41	F	L	29.7	1320	6.0
JD	20	38	M	L	15.6	1020	8.6†
KC	20	22	M	C	16.1	615	9.8
MF	20	20	M	L	—	635	5.6†
CB	20	44	F	L	31.4	647	8.6†
GR	20	35	M	L	23.2	1154	10.1*
AS	20	48	M	L	11.6	633	5.9‡

Source of donor kidney is indicated by L (living related) or C (of cadaveric origin). Normal values for the laboratory are urea 2.5–6.7 mmol/1; creatinine 70–150 μmol/l; haemoglobin 14–18 g/dl. Other intercurrent medication is * = cimetidine/ranitidine; † = B-adrenoreceptor drugs; ‡ = hydralazine. The mean weight was 61.1 kg, range 41–82 kg. Operation time was about 160 minutes and blood loss less than 200 ml. For all patients the plasma concentration of bilirubin and activity of aspartate aminotransferase were within normal limits.

plasma was stored frozen until analysis. Sampling times were up to 180 minutes in all patients, and to 1440 minutes in seven patients (six having 20 mg and one 10 mg morphine sulphate). The donor kidney was a living related transplant in eight patients, and of cadaveric origin in the remaining seven.

Control patients

Two control groups were used, one to provide plasma morphine concentrations over 24 hours and the other as controls for the anaesthetic effects alone. None of the control patients had any renal, hepatic or cardiovascular disease, nor were they receiving any regular medication known to interfere with morphine kinetics. Control data for intraoperative morphine kinetics up to three hours was obtained from 14 patients undergoing lumbar laminectomy. They received a similar anaesthetic to the transplant group, and were given 10 mg morphine sulphate intravenously. Control data to 24 hours was obtained from five awake patients with chronic pain given 20 mg morphine sulphate intravenously.

Analytical methods

Plasma morphine was measured by specific radioimmunoassay (Moore *et al.* 1984*a*). To exclude interference in the morphine radioimmunoassay, morphine was also measured by liquid chromatography (Moore *et al.* 1984*b*) with extraction, ion-paired reverse-phase chromatography and amperometric detection. Plasma creatinine and urea were measured by a standard procedure using an IL 919 analyser.

For those patients with 24-hour data, the area under the concentration time curve (AUC) for morphine was determined by the trapezoidal method. Plasma clearance for 24 hours was calculated from the formula:

$$\text{Clearance} = \text{Dose}/\text{AUC}_{0-24h}.$$

Terminal half-life for morphine was estimated by linear regression analysis using sample points after the plateau phase

Plasma concentrations of morphine from the control groups were compared with those from patients undergoing transplantation at various sampling times using the Mann–Whitney 'U' test. This test was also used to compare the calculated clearance and terminal half-life values. Changes in plasma morphine concentration with time, and morphine concentrations measured by both radioimmunoassay and liquid chromatography were compared using the paired 't' test.

Results

There was an initial rapid fall in the plasma morphine concentrations for both the 15 transplant patients and 14 anaesthetized control subjects over the first 10 minutes and in the control subjects the plasma morphine concentration continued to decline. Between 20 and 180 minutes this fall was statistically significant ($p < 0.01$, paired 't' test) for controls. However, there was no significant change in plasma morphine concentrations in the transplant group between 20 and 180 minutes. Dose-corrected plasma morphine concentrations were significantly higher in transplant patients than in the controls at all sample times after 30 minutes ($p < 0.05$, Mann–Whitney 'U' test).

Figure 3 shows individual plasma morphine concentrations over 24 hours for six transplant patients given 20 mg morphine compared with mean plasma morphine concentations from the five awake controls. The duration of the plateau phase in the five living related donor transplants was about five hours. Thereafter plasma morphine declined in a similar manner to the controls. In the single patient shown who received a cadaveric transplant, plasma morphine remained elevated for a considerable period, declining slowly over the first two postoperative days. Plasma morphine concentrations for the living related donors were significantly ($p < 0.01$) greater than in the controls between 2 and 12 hours after injection.

The calculated kinetic parameters for both transplant and 24-hour controls are shown in Table 3. The 24-hour AUC and the calculated 24-hour plasma clearance for the transplant patients were significantly different from those of the controls ($p < 0.01$). However, there was no significant difference for the calculated terminal half-life between controls (mean 224 minutes, range 120–350) and living related transplants (mean 236 minutes, range 150–280).

In those transplant patients where samples were obtained for 24 hours, plasma creatinine was also measured. In each patient the plasma creatinine concentration was constant for about five hours after the dose of morphine; thereafter it fell over the remaining observation period. A significant change from the plateau concentration was defined as more than the twice the intra-assay coefficient of variation. In each patient the point at which the plasma creatinine fell significantly was the point at which plasma morphine also fell significantly.

Nineteen plasma samples obtained during the plateau phase from five transplant patients were analysed by both radioimmunoassay and by a liquid chromatographic

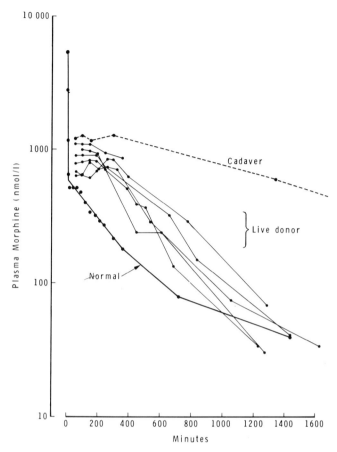

Fig. 3. Mean plasma morphine concentrations for five non-anaesthetized control subjects and individual values for six transplant patients to about 24 hours after injection. All received 20 mg morphine sulphate i.v.

method. There were no statistically significant or systematic differences between the two methods, and mean values for these samples were similar (786 nmol/l for radioimmunoassay, compared with 802 nmol/l for chromatography).

Discussion

Morphine kinetics were altered during renal transplantation. The prolonged period during which morphine concentrations did not fall, both during anaesthesia and after the operation, was solely responsible for the increased AUC and decreased morphine clearance, because the terminal morphine half-life in the living related transplants was the same as in the controls.

The plateau was not due to anaesthesia or anaesthetic drugs, because the transplant patients received a similar anaesthetic to the anaesthetised controls, in whom no prolonged plateau in morphine concentration was seen. The possibility that the prolonged plateau phase was due to cross-reactivity with accumulating morphine

Table 3
Calculated kinetic parameters for transplant and control patients

Patient	AUC$_{0-24}$ (nmol. min/l)	Clearance (ml/min)	Clearance per kg (ml/min/kg)	Terminal half-life (min)
Transplant				
MC	439 694	120	2.02	230
GR	544 974	97	1.18	280
AS	469 093	113	1.60	270
CB	535 995	99	1.61	270
GF	443 490	119	2.40	220
KC*	1 919 773	28	0.53	740
PC†	206 360	128	3.12	150
Mean	486 649‡	101	1.78	236§
SD	50 529	34	0.84	48
Control				
A	167 540	315	4.4	210
B	180 340	293	4.6	170
C	235 050	225	3.3	120
D	267 280	197	2.9	350
E	287 530	184	2.7	270
Mean	227 548	243	3.58	224
SD	52 588	58	0.87	89

All transplant patients had living related donor kidneys and were given 20 mg morphine sulphate except * (cadaveric donor) and † (10 mg morphine sulphate). For the transplant group, mean AUC (‡) omits data from both these patients and mean terminal half-life (§) omits data from patient with cadaveric graft. There was no significant difference between the groups for terminal half-life. The plasma morphine clearance for all transplant patients against controls was significantly lower ($p = 0.002$), as it was for living related donors only ($p = 0.009$).

metabolites is unlikely; the radioimmunoassay correlated well with a high-performance liquid chromatography method for samples from the plateau phase.

These results suggest that the removal of morphine from the body was not dependent solely upon hepatic extraction and metabolism. In the transplant patients (who had normal preoperative hepatic function, as judged by liver enzyme and bilirubin measurements) plasma morphine concentrations plateaued between about 500 and 1000 nmol/l. This implied that no appreciable hepatic extraction was occurring. Evidence to support the role of the kidney in morphine removal was seen in the simultaneous onset of the decline in plasma creatinine and morphine concentrations. Plasma creatinine will begin to fall when kidney function has recovered following the period of cold ischaemia. For the single patient receiving a cadaveric graft, return of renal function occurred more slowly due to the prolonged period of cold ischaemia; the fall in both plasma creatinine and plasma morphine was delayed.

Biochemical evidence suggests that the kidney may be more important in morphine elimination than had been appreciated. The rabbit proximal tubule is able to accumulate morphine and metabolize the drug to its glucuronides at concentrations of 700 nmol/l (Schali and Roch-Ramel 1982), in contrast to the Michaelis constant for morphine glucuronidation in human liver microsomes of 1,000,000 nmol/l (Sawe *et al.*

1982). In cirrhotic patients with normal renal function no difference was found in the clearance of morphine compared with volunteers (Patwardhan *et al.* 1981). While both the liver and kidney are involved in morphine metabolism, the kidney may be relatively more important at plasma concentrations in the therapeutic range. The evidence from the unique circumstance of the transplantation of a normal kidney to patients with impaired renal function supports this. The implication for clinical practice is that morphine should be administered with caution to patients with renal insufficiency.

Acknowledgements

We wish to thank Professor P. J. Morris for allowing us to study his patients, the patients for their co-operation, and the anaesthetic and renal unit staff for their help. This study was supported by the Medical Research Council and the Oxford Regional Health Authority. Preliminary results were presented at a meeting on 'Opioid analgesics in the management of clinical pain' held at memorial Sloan-Kettering Cancer Centre, New York, in July 1983.

References

Baird, G. D., Symonds, H. W., and Ash, R. (1975). Some observations on metabolite production and utilisation *in vivo* by the gut and liver of adult dairy cows. *J. agric. Sci.* **85,** 281.

Bartlett, A. J., Lloyd-Jones, J. G., Rance, M. J., Flockhart, I. R., Dockray, G. J., Bennett, M. R. D., and Moore, R. A. (1980). The radioimmunoassay of bupre-norphine. *Eur. J. clin. Pharmacol.* **18,** 339.

Bullingham, R. E. S., McQuay, H. J., Porter, E. J. B., Thomas, D., Allen, M. C., and Moore, R. A. (1982). Acute i.v. methadone kinetics in man: relationship to chronic studies. *Br. J. Anaesth.* **54,** 1271.

McQuay, H. J., Moore, R. A., Paterson, G. M. C., and Adams, A. P. (1979). Plasma fentanyl concentrations and clinical observations during and after operation. *Br. J. Anaesth.* **51,** 543.

Moore, R. A., Baldwin, D., Allen, M. C., Watson, P. J. Q., Bullingham, R. E. S., and McQuay, H. J. (1984*a*). Sensitive and specific morphine radioimmunoassay with iodine label: pharmacokinetics of morphine in man after intravenous admini-stration. *Annls clin. Biochem.*, in press.

——— McQuay, H. J., and Bullingham, R. E. S. (1984*b*). HPLC of morphine with electrochemical detection: analysis in human plasma. *Annls clin. Biochem.* in press.

Patwardhan, R. V., Johnson, R. F., Hoyumpa, A., Sheehan, J. J., Desmond, P. V., Wilkinson, G. R., Branch, R. A., and Schenker, S. (1981). Normal metabolism of morphine in cirrhosis. *Gastroenterology* **81,** 1006.

Sawe, J., Dahlstrom, B., Paalzow, L., and Rane, A. (1981). Morphine kinetics in cancer patients. *Clin. Pharmacol. Ther.* **30,** 629.

——— Pacifici, G. M., Kager, L., von Bahr, C., and Rane, A. (1982). Glucuronidation of morphine in human liver and interaction with oxazepam. *Acta anaesth. scand.* Suppl. **74,** 47.

Schali, C. and Roch-Ramel, F. (1982). Transport and metabolism of [³H]-morphine in isolated, nonperfused proximal tubular segments of the rabbit kidney. *J. Pharmacol. exp. Ther.* **223,** 811.

Stanski, D. R., Greenblatt, D. J., Lappas, D. G., Kock-Weser, J., and Lowenstein, E. (1976).

Kinetics of high-dose intravenous morphine in cardiac surgery patients. *Clin. Pharmacol. Ther.* **19**, 752.

Symonds, H. W. and Baird, G. D. (1973). Cannulation of an hepatic vein, the portal vein and a mesenteric vein in the cow, and its use in the measurement of blood flow rates. *Res. vet. Sci.* **14**, 267.

MST Continus tablets in pain of advanced cancer: a controlled study

H. HENRIKSEN and JULIE KNUDSEN

Department of Anaesthesia,
Finsen Institute,
Copenhagen,
Denmark

In the Finsen Institute (a cancer hospital, 250 beds) one of our methods of treating severe pain is morphine chloride tablets given four-hourly. Recently MST Continus tablets (Napp Laboratories Ltd.) 12-hourly have been introduced. The aim of this study was to compare the results of the two ways of morphine administration.

Material

Sixteen patients with pain due to metastatic or invasive cancer were studied. The patients were in advanced stages, but not terminal. All patients were on long-term morphine treatment, and had been so for at least eight days. Their daily dose at entrance to the study had been constant for at least eight days. The data are shown in Table 1.

Method

The study design is shown in Fig. 1. The patients were randomized to a cross-over sequence so that all patients received morphine chloride four-hourly for one week and MST 12-hourly for one week. The pattern of tablet intake was the same in both weeks (i.e. four-hourly), because placebo tablets were included. Medication times were 10 a.m. and 10 p.m. for MST and 10 a.m., 2 p.m., 6 p.m. and 10 p.m., 2 a.m., 6 a.m. for morphine chloride.

Measurements consisted of visual analogue scale (VAS) ratings for pain and sedation every two hours between 10 a.m. and 10 p.m. on all 14 study days.

After week 2, the patients were interviewed about their preference for week 1 or week 2.

Side effects and the use of rescue analgesics were recorded.

Advances in Morphine Therapy. The 1983 International Symposium on Pain Control, edited by E. Wilkes, 1984: Royal Society of Medicine International Congress and Symposium Series No. 64, published by the Royal Society of Medicine.

Table 1

Patient Data

No.	Sex	Age	Previous morphine HCl treatment	
			duration (days)	daily dose (mg) at entrance
1	F	47	14	180
2	F	56	16	180
3	M	56	84	270
4	F	47	15	60
5	F	61	42	270
6	F	66	28	360
7	F	65	21	120
8	M	39	8	360
9	M	44	42	360
10	M	38	136	540
11	F	54	14	60
12	F	53	42	270
13	F	65	9	270
14	M	60	21	90
15	M	64	28	360
16	F	47	42	360

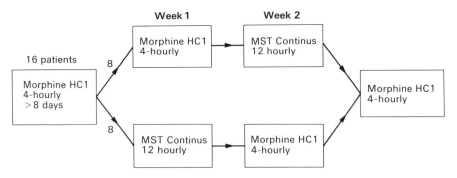

Measurements: Pain VAS daily at 0, 2, 4, 6, 8, 10, 12 h.
Sedation VAS daily at 0, 2, 4, 6, 8, 10, 12h
Assessments: Patient preference for Week 1/Week 2
Side-effects
Rescue analgesics

Fig. 1. Design of study.

Results

As shown in Fig. 2 the mean pain VAS values of the 16 patients in seven days were close to 20 mm with no statistically significant difference between the two preparations. Only at 12 hours a slight trend towards a higher pain score in the MST week was found. The mean value of all observations was 22.2 for MST and 20.9 for morphine chloride. This difference has no clinical importance.

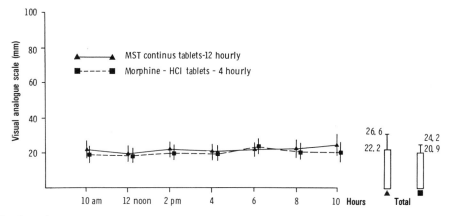

Fig. 2. Pain scores in oral morphine treatment in advanced cancer (mean of 16 patients
(±SEM) in seven days).

Figure 3 shows the VAS scores for sedation. There is a slight difference at 10 and 12
hours. This difference originates only from the first three days (during which the
difference was statistically significant), whereas there was no difference in the last four
days. The mean value of all observations was 13.7 for MST and 11.8 for morphine
chloride.

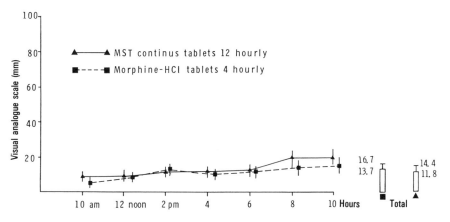

Fig. 3. Sedation scores in oral morphine treatment in advanced cancer (mean of 16 patients
(±SEM) in seven days).

Patient preference

Five of the 16 patients had no preference for either week. Eight patients preferred the
week with morphine chloride four-hourly, three patients preferred the week with MST
12-hourly. However, of the 11 patients who did have a preference, 10 patients preferred
the first week, no matter which drug was given. It was also noted that patient
preferences were not in accordance with their actual pain scoring.

Rescue analgesics

The use of extra analgesics (paracetamol or ibuprofen) was very modest and not significantly different in the two weeks.

Side-effects

Eight patients had no incidence of nausea and vomiting in either week. Seven patients reported 12 incidences of nausea and vomiting in the MST week, 14 incidences in the morphine chloride week. One patient reported a lot of nausea and vomiting in both weeks, but most in the MST week. Eight patients reported no incidence of dizziness, seven patients reported dizziness at 21 scoring times in MST week and two scoring times in morphine chloride week. Again one patient had a lot of dizziness but most in the MST week.

   We think that in this study there was no significant difference between side-effects of the two preparations, but a statistical analysis would require a much larger patient series.

Summary

In a double-blind cross-over study we have found equally good relief of pain of advanced cancer with MST Continus tablets given every 12 hours and with conventional morphine chloride tablets given every four hours, provided that the total dose is the same. Sedation was slightly greater with MST, but only during the first three days of MST intake. The other side-effects were similar.

The 1983 International Symposium on Pain Control

Summary of the day

D. VERE

What I might do perhaps just very briefly is to refer to a few punch lines which seem to me to have come out. Subjective measures are indeed respectable scientifically, but it has been very important today to have the patients mental state emphasized, especially the effects of depression. The discussion then broadened into the whole area of quality of life, and also into the area of tests in analgesic therapy of severe pain in the clinical context in the last two weeks of life, and also before that. I must say I would not feel worried about a test being made just within the last two weeks of life. In fact I feel very encouraged that people have invaded this extremely difficult territory and are beginning to produce helpful data about these problems. I am a little disturbed about to-day's title 'intractable pain control' because I do not know what your experience has been, but mine has been that intractable pain is usually synonymous with failed opiate management. Truly intractable pain is very rare although we have heard about one or two distressing cases to-day. These cases exist. We must not run away from that conclusion, but they are far, far less frequent than is imagined by the general medical populace. What I think we have not perhaps sufficiently clarified is a presentation of treatment to the patient in terms of pain tolerance on the one hand, and pain removal on the other, and related these two very different goals to pain perception on the part of the individual patient. This is an area in which I think there is a great deal of work to be done in advanced methodology.

I am not going to talk any more about the vexed issue of the relationship of pain relief to plasma morphine levels, but just to underscore the points that have already been made to-day. Morphine assays are still in a stage of evolution; they have improved enormously over the time when most of the work that has been presented and discussed here has been done. Radioimmunoassays I think are acceptable in certain situations and certain methods, but do need to be viewed with particular criticism because of the problem of metabolites and cross-reacting drugs which may be present in the patient in addition to morphine. We must be very, very critical about assays in that field and I do not doubt that the radioimmunoassays can be made satisfactory.

Napp Laboratories had a conference very recently about the whole problem of morphine assays and this is published (Stuart 1983) and I think it is a very important

Advances in Morphine Therapy. The 1983 International Symposium on Pain Control, edited by E. Wilkes, 1984: Royal Society of Medicine International Congress and Symposium Series No. 64, published by the Royal Society of Medicine.

contribution to that field of discussion. We must not forget also thinking about pharmacokinetic sequestration. Pethidine sequests in the stomach in chalk nitrogen containing molecules and morphine probably does so to a lesser extent. That is just one example of a sort of sequestration which can occur. We must be very much aware of this. Now I think we have this very important question raised in to-day's papers; 'Is the classical pharmacokinetic pattern that we have all been taught for morphine in fact correct?' Does extrahepatic metabolism occur?

I must say I enjoyed very much the quote which I shall treasure that 'enterohepatic recirculation is an old chestnut which keeps coming back'. That is certainly worth repetition.

Someone referred to the question of old drugs being rehashed; and I must say that when I heard that I thought, 'no, not really'. I believe that if you put an old drug into a new formulation it really behaves like a new drug in some ways, and needs to be thought about as if it were, at least with some sort of critical and sensitive approach. I think that Napp Laboratories Ltd., being pioneers of controlled-release preparations in this field, have really bitten off a very large area of—shall I say educational difficulty. We have large numbers of doctors who were trained either before the Second World War or shortly afterwards. They were brought up in the comfortable atmosphere of using a drug several times a day which would just give the patient a sniff of benefit and then safety as it was quickly removed from the body. If we are going to use controlled-release drugs by mouth, if we are going to use syringe drivers and epidural administration, we are in a different ball park and we dare not treat that sort of therapy in the old-fashioned ways that our medical and nursing professions are so familiar with: there will be a lot of false security if we do.

We need to teach new sets of attitudes and this is something you might say is for the medical educators to do, but it is so difficult to reach so many of the people who are handling drugs in actual medical practice. Napp Laboratories have helped in this area by organizing such a Symposium as this one.

On the question of trials, I do not think that there are severe problems in cross-over trials in short-lived patients beyond those that have already been described. Those exist and they are very important, but I think they throw into relief a very important attitude to trials which perhaps is not conventional. Trials are made in large groups of people which contain numerous subpopulations and the modern attitude of clinical trial design is very much a 'horses for courses' approach as we call it in England. We try to individuate towards small groups of patients even to single individuals within groups. This makes statistics very difficult, but it has to be done and I think the hospice trials have thrown this into relief that there is a subgroup that you can take into a trial and look at critically, and that there are other very real and very important patients who pose problems, but I would just repeat the point that I made earlier that provided those problems are balanced between treatment groups they do not invalidate the trial. What I think is very important is the point that Michael Baum raised about small numbers and the beta-error—the type-two error that is extremely important, because if the outcome of your study is going to be that there is no detectable difference, then the beta-error comes into its own as extremely important. We also need to define very carefully what biological differences we would regard as important.

It was very interesting to hear Richard Lamerton discussing the hospice or hospital–home interface. What an important area that is and it needs a lot more close discussion, and that leads me on to just mention very briefly things which I do not think we have discussed sufficiently yet—respiratory depression.

I am concerned at the concern so many people still have about this problem. I think that the sort of questions we should be asking about a drug like MST Continus tablets is, does the controlled-release system avoid the problems of nausea and vomiting?

Does it avoid the need to keep to rigid times of administration, and so on? But, respiratory depression—no. I saw a patient recently who was accidentally given a tenfold overdose of MST Continus tablets, but so long as I kept talking to him he remained awake, and at the end of about six hours he said, 'You know this is wonderful—this is the first time that my pain is relieved since I have been in here'. It is not the problem that so many people take it for and so please let us educate one another and others out of this paranoid worry about respiratory depression. How can we persuade surgeons that patients which have 'n' operations which have failed. The probability of an $n + 1$ operation helping them is exceedingly small—perhaps 0.5 to the n. Very little chance that some surgery will help.

Those were the punch lines to me. You will no doubt have others.

Reference

Stuart, J. F. B. (ed.) (1983). *Methods of morphine estimation in biological fluids and the concept of free morphine*. Royal Society of Medicine International Congress and Symposium Series No. 58. Royal Society of Medicine/Academic Press, London.

The treatment of pain in terminal illness

J. LEVY et al.

Napp Laboratories Ltd.,
Cambridge

Introduction

Terminal illness is defined as 'a state of disease characterized by a progressive deterioration with impairment of function and survival limited in time, usually from several days to a few months'. In England and Wales approximately 130 000 people die each year from neoplastic disease (Mortality Statistics 1981). Their terminal illness is characterized by a variety of symptoms which may include pain, anorexia, nausea, vomiting, insomnia, dyspnoea, coughing, anxiety, depression, and mental confusion. Relief of these symptoms is embodied in the concept of 'dying with dignity' (Vanderpool 1978). In the terminally ill this means the control of the patient's own fate rather than endurance of the indignities of an incurable disease in its terminal stages and the maintenance of as much self-esteem as possible. Thus 'caring' is considered as important as 'curing'. Since drugs are self-administered, they involve the patient in his own treatment and reduce the patient's dependency on the clinic or the physician.

In the care of the terminally ill, drugs used should maximize patient comfort. Unnecessary diagnostic procedures and treatment should be avoided. The patient and not the disease becomes the target for care and treatment of the symptoms becomes the prime objective.

Pain relief in terminal neoplasia is mainly achieved by narcotic analgesics. Dextromoramide (Twycross 1978) and pethidine (Marks and Sachar 1973) have the disadvantage that they both have a very short duration of action. This is an obvious disadvantage in the treatment of continuous pain. Methadone has the disadvantage of a very long plasma half-life (Verebely *et al.* 1975; Nilsson *et al.* 1982) which may result in life-threatening accumulation (Leslie *et al.* 1977; Ettinger *et al.* 1979; Berkowitz 1976). Methadone also has a sedative action which considerably outlasts its analgesic activity. Morphine formulated in MST Continus tablets (Napp Laboratories Ltd.) is considered the treatment of choice (Clarke 1982). In the treatment of pain, administration must avoid the onset of pain rather than administration on a patient-request basis. Physicians often choose the latter because of concern for addiction, but this is not a consideration in the terminally ill as treatment is for a limited duration. In practice, addiction does not occur with short-term treatment and patients on longer-term

Advances in Morphine Therapy. The 1983 International Symposium on Pain Control, edited by E. Wilkes, 1984: Royal Society of Medicine International Congress and Symposium Series No. 64, published by the Royal Society of Medicine.

treatment have even experienced dosage reduction. Since the pain is continuous, rational treatment requires administration in such a way as to maintain analgesic levels continuously. The Continus mechanism achieves continual maintenance of analgesia on a simple twice-daily dosage regimen (Welsh *et al.* 1983). Time-contingent administration has the advantage of dissociating pain and drug administration and reduces the anxiety and fear associated with anticipation of pain.

Morphine helps control other symptoms associated with neoplastic disease such as coughing and dyspnoea. MST Continus tablets may also reduce the sedative requirement for insomnia since pain relief is extended throughout the night preventing sleep disturbance. Pain relief also allays anxiety and depression and this may also indirectly reduce insomnia.

Adjunctive treatment of pain may also be achieved by radiotherapy, surgery, hormonal treatment, and chemotherapy of the disease itself. Elevation of the pain threshold is produced by treatment with antidepressants, corticosteroids, and non-steroidal anti-inflammatory agents. The latter may enhance analgesia by prevention of prostaglandin release and reduction of the inflammatory process. Release of prostaglandin release and reduction of the inflammatory process. Release of prostaglandin is thought to contribute to pain particularly in patients with skeletal metastasis.

In order to increase patient compliance and reduce the daily tablet burden MST Continus tablets were introduced at the two higher dosage strengths, namely, 60 and 100 mg and the two dosage forms were investigated in two multi-centre open clinical trials.

Investigators

E. Allen, Christie Hospital, Withington, Manchester.

R. E. Atkinson, Royal Hospital, Chesterfield, Derbyshire.

V. L. Barley, Radiotherapy and Oncology Centre, Horfield Road, Bristol.

I. M. C. Clarke, North West Pain Relief Centre, Hope Hospital, Salford.

N. Cole, Pain Clinic, District General Hospital, Eastbourne, Sussex.

J. Croudace, Compton Hall Ltd., Compton, Wolverhampton.

R. J. Dickson, Michael Sobell House, Mount Vernon Hospital, Northwood, Middlesex.

C. Greaves, St. Luke's Nursing Home, Sheffield.

G. M. Halliday, St. Columba's Hospice, Edinburgh.

J. Hester, Pain Clinic, District General Hospital, Eastbourne, Sussex.

J. Hunton, South Cleveland Hospital, Middlesbrough, Cleveland.

E. P. Johnson, St. Bartholomew's Hospital, Rochester, Kent.

R. A. Lyons, Mount Edgcumbe Hospice, St. Austell, Cornwall.

I. M. M. Macmillan, Ladywell Medical Centre, Edinburgh.

W. Macrae, Ninewells Hospital, Dundee.

D. G. Morgan, Royal Berkshire Hospital, Reading, Berks.

A. Naysmith, Department of Oncology, The Middlesex Hospital, London

A. L. G. Peel, North Tees General Hospital, Hardwick, Stockton on Tees, Cleveland.

Colonel N. Peters, Queen Elizabeth Military Hospital, Woolwich, London.

L. R. Redman, Royal United Hospital, Bath, Avon.

C. C. Spanswick, Department of Anaesthesia, Park Hospital, Manchester.

G. A. Stone, St. Luke's Nursing Home, Sheffield.

R. Twycross, Sir Michael Sobell House, The Churchill Hospital, Headington, Oxford.

C. Wood, Oncology Department, Hackney Hospital, London.

Study A

A multi-centre evaluation of MST Continus tablets 60 mg in the treatment of pain in terminal illness.

Patients and methods

A multi-centre clinical trial was carried out in 15 centres to determine the efficacy of MST Continus tablets 60 mg in the treatment of patients with pain due to terminal neoplastic disease. The participating physicians completed questionnaires to provide the patient data for this study.

Sixty-seven patients (35 male and 32 female) age 26–78 years entered an open clinical trial. The mean age of the patients was 57.6 years.

The primary site of the neoplasm, where known, is shown in Table 1. The predominant diagnoses were carcinoma of the breast and lung. Twenty-five patients had metastatic disease, mainly skeletal.

Table 1

Primary site of the neoplasm

Neoplasm site	No. of patients
Lung	14
Cervix	8
Rectum	7
Prostate	5
Breast	12
Pancreas	2
Caecum	2
Floor of mouth	2
Ovary	1
Bladder	1
Parotid	1
Kidney (transitional cell)	1
Oropharynx	1
Nasopharynx	1
Multiple myeloma	1
Osteosarcoma (lower limb)	1
Malignant schwannoma	1
Unknown primary site	6

Table 2

Previous drug treatment

Treatment	No. of patients
MST Continus tablets 10 and 30 mg	27
DF118	6
Distalgesic	6
Buprenorphine	5
Diamorphine	9
Diconal	5
Morphine	2
Pethidine	7
Zomepirac	1
Brompton mixture	2
Diflunisal	5
Dextromoramide	4
Paramol-118	1
Isocarboxazid	1
Papaveretum	1
Pentazocine	1
Cocaine elixir	1
Garlic tablets	1
Aspirin	1
Methadone	1
Morphine mix	10
Phenazocine	3
Haloperidol	1
Triptafen-DA	1

Previous drug treatment is shown in Table 2 and additional drugs received by the patients are listed in Table 3.

MST Continus tablets 60 mg were given at a dosage titrated for each patient to produce continual pain relief. The dosage regimen, the total daily dosage, tablet number, and duration of treatment was recorded. Any incidence of pain breakthrough during treatment with MST Continus tablets 60 mg was treated with additional analgesics and their use was noted.

During the patient's last few days of life some became unable to swallow tablets. Other analgesics and the alternative routes of administration in these cases were recorded.

Results and discussion

During treatment with MST Continus tablets 60 mg, the total daily dose of morphine given ranged from 60 to 720 mg/day with a mean value of 244 mg/day. The mean daily tablet number was four tablets/day. Treatment was given twice daily in 39 patients and three times daily in 24; it was administered every six hours in one patient and the frequency was unspecified in three. The patients received MST Continus tablets 60 mg for 2–365 days (mean 38 days). For 61 patients in whom the dosage duration was specified, it represents 2253 patient-days of treatment.

Table 3

Concurrent medication

Antiphlogistics (19)	*Cytostatics (3)*
Flurbiprofen 9	Tamoxifen 1
Diflunisal 3	Aminoglutethimide 1
Indomethacin 2	Estramustine 1
Benorylate 4	
Ibuprofen 1	*Sedatives (4)*
	Diazepam 2
Corticosteroids (11)	Temazepam 1
Prednisolone 6	Ketazolam 1
Dexamethasone 4	
Cortisone 1	*Other Drugs (19)*
	Frusemide 3
Laxatives (6)	Potassium Chloride 2
Dorbanex 6	Oxymetholone 1
	Codeine 1
Phenothiazines (5)	Benylin 1
Chorpromazine 3	Temazepam 3
Prochlorperazine 2	Haloperidol 2
	Buprenorphine 1
Antidepressants (7)	Digoxin 1
Mianserin 3	Warfarin 1
Triptafen-DA 3	Aminophylline 2
Amitriptyline 1	Metronidazole 1

The clinician's assessment of the pain-relief response was classified on a scale from 0 to 4 as indicated in Table 4.

Good/excellent responses were achieved in 46/63 (73 per cent) patients; 63 per cent on a twice-daily dosage regimen and 91 per cent on a thrice-daily dosage regimen.

There was no obvious dose–response relationship. Patients with a poor response received a similar mean dosage to those with an excellent response and the poor responders were almost entirley confined to those on a twice-daily dosage regimen. This suggests that some patients with severe pain may require more frequent administration. They may represent a group of rapid metabolizers of morphine.

Fifteen patients required additional analgesia. One patient required palfium on two occasions and another required additional analgesia rarely. In one patient also given cyclimorph, intrathecal diamorphine had failed to control his pain. Two patients were unable to swallow tablets just before their death.

Table 4

Pain relief response assessment

Response score	Clinician's assessment
0	Deterioration
1	Inadequate pain control
2	Moderate pain control
3	Good pain control
4	Complete pain relief

Table 5

Patient response in relation to total daily dosage and dosage frequency

Pain relief score	No. of patients	Daily dosage frequency			MST-60 daily dosage (mg/day)	
		twice	thrice	N/A	Mean	Range
0	5	4	0	1	270	120–480
1	6*	4	1	—	250	120–480
2	6	5	1	—	210	120–360
3	33	11	20	2	233	60–540
4	13	11	1	1	240	120–720
N/A	4	3	1	—	235	100–360

* One four times a day administration.

Side-effects

MST Continus tablets were well tolerated. Several patients commented on the lack of side-effects and relief from anorexia produced by the preparation. Side-effects of nausea and constipation did not present as a problem in this study possibly because of the concurrent treatment with laxatives and antiemetics. Habituation did not present as a problem in this study. In fact dosage reduction was possible in one patient and another patient managed with a lower dose following palliative radiotherapy.

Conclusion

MST Continus tablets 60 mg were well tolerated and showed good efficacy in the treatment of pain in terminal neoplasia. Anlaysis of the data suggested that poor responders may benefit from a thrice-daily rather than a twice-daily dosage regimen or an increase in the twice-daily dosage.

Study B

A multi-centre evaluation of MST Continus tablets 100 mg in the treatment of pain in terminal illness.

Patients and methods

Clinical investigators from 21 centres entered patients with severe pain due to terminal neoplasia into an open trial of MST Continus tablets 100 mg. The trial design followed that of the 60 mg tablet and its purpose was to investigate the efficacy of the 100 mg formulation.

Forty-eight patients (20 male and 28 female) aged 25–80 years entered the study. The mean patient age was 56.4 years. The patients' diagnosis is shown in Table 6. Thirty patients had metastatic disease. Previous analgesic treatment is shown in Table 7 and

Table 6

Primary site of the neoplasm

Neoplasm site	No. of patients
Breast	11
Lung	12
Rectum	4
Kidney	2
Prostate	4
Cervix	3
Bladder	3
Thyroid	1
Pharynx	1
Ovary	1
Floor of mouth	1
Sigmoid colon	2
Lymphoblastic lymphoma	1
Sarcoma femur	1
Wegener's granulomatosis	1

Table 7

Previous analgesic treatment

Treatment	No. of patients
Diamorphine	10
Morphine	9
DF118	6
MST Continus tablets 60 mg	4
MST Continus tablets 30 mg	4
MST Continus tablets 10 mg	3
Phenazocine	3
Distalgesic	4
Dextromoramide	8
Buprenorphine	3
Brompton cocktail	2
Pentazocine	1
Diconal	3
Pethidine	2
Aqueous chloroform	1
Cosalgesic	1
Paracetamol	1
Disprin	1
Codis	1
Alcohol	1
Indomethacin	1

Table 8

Concurrent treatment

Corticosteroids (23)	*Cytostatics (12)*
Prednisolone 12	Tamoxifen 6
Dexamethasone 6	Fosfestrol 1
Betamethasone 2	Nandrolone 1
Prednisone 1	Medroxyprogesterone 1
Fludrocortisone 1	Aminoglutethimide 1
Cortisone 1	Diethylstilboestrol 1
	Azathioprine 1
Sedatives (8)	
Lorazepam 2	*Antidepressants (8)*
Temazepam 2	Amitriptyline 3
Flurazepam 1	Unspecified 1
Diazepam 3	Triptafen-DA 1
	Mianserin 2
Laxatives (14)	Dothiepin 1
Dorbanex 8	
Lactulose 5	*Antiphlogistics (12)*
Bisacodyl 1	Indomethacin 3
	Diflunisal 6
Phenothiazines (9)	Phenylbutazone 2
Chlorpromazine 1	Flurbiprofen 1
Prochlorperzine 8	
	Others (18)
	Bendrofluazide 2
	Haloperidol 3
	Clonazepam 1
	Domperidone 1

concurrent treatment is listed in Table 8. It is interesting to note that patients were co-prescribed from one to ten additional drugs.

Results and discussion

The majority of patients (35) received MST Continus tablets 100 mg on a twice-daily dosage regimen while 11 received treatment three times daily. One patient received treatment every six hours. The mean daily dosage was 415 mg/day (range 200–1600 mg/day) for 47 patients. The mean duration of treatment was 45 days (range 4–222 days) and for 47 patients this represented 2135 patient-days of treatment.

The patient's response was available in 46 patients and was converted to a digital score. Good/excellent responses were reported for 39/46 patients (84 per cent). A good response was achieved at a mean morphine dose of 423 mg/day (number of patients = 25) while an excellent response was achieved in 18 patients at a mean daily dose of 455 mg/day (see Table 9).

Twenty-two patients occasionally required additional analgesia. They received diamorphine (ten), morphine (three), distalgesic (two), dextromoramide (one), aspirin (three), cosalgesic (two), parcetamol (one), and DF118 (two). Two further patients occasionally needed DF118 and morphine.

The mean daily dosage of MST Continus tablets 100 mg in 23 patients with 'escape analgesia' was 419 mg/day.

Table 9

Patient response in relation to total daily dosage and dosage frequency

Pain relief score	No. of patients	Daily dosage frequency			MST-100 dosage (mg/day)	
		twice	thrice	N/A	Mean	Range
0	1	—	1	—	300	—
1	0	—	—	—	—	—
2	2	2	—	—	230	200–260
3	25*	18	5	1	423	200–1100
4	18	14	4	—	455	200–1600
N/A	2	2	—	—	200	—

* One four times a day administration.

Five patients became unable to swallow tablets on their last few days before death and were given diamorphine solution orally, morphine or morphine suppositories.

Side-effects

MST Continus tablets 100 mg were well tolerated. The usual side-effects of transient nausea and constipation associated with opiate analgesics were not observed in this study as patients were correctly prescribed routine laxatives and antiemetics. One patient experienced drowsiness and slight nausea for the first 2–3 days of treatment. Otherwise all patients remained mentally alert and relatively active. There was no instance of habituation.

Conclusion

MST Continus tablets 100 mg provide good continuous relief from pain in patients with terminal neoplasia. They allow treatment on a simple twice-daily dosage schedule and are effective throughout the night. They allow treatment on a simple twice-daily dosage schedule and are effective throughout the night. They allow undisturbed sleep since patients do not have to be woken to be given analgesic treatment. The tablets were extremely well tolerated and this together with their efficacy and small size encourages patient compliance.

References

Berkowitz, B. A. (1976). The relationship of pharmacokinetics to pharmacologic activity: morphine, methadone and naloxone. *Clin. Pharmacokinet.* **1,** 219.

Clarke, I. M. C. (1982). Old drugs for old aches. *Update* **24,** 2297.

Ettinger, D. S., Vitale, P. J., and Trump, D. L. (1979). Important clinical pharmacological considerations in the use of methadone in cancer patients. *Cancer Treat. Rep.* **63,** 457.

Leslie, S. T., Miller, R. B., and Boroda, C. (1977). Methadone: evidence of accumulation. *Br. med. J.* **i,** 375.

Marks, R. M., and Sachar, E. J. (1973). Undertreatment of medical inpatients with narcotic analgesics. *Ann. intern. Med.* **78,** 173.

Mortality Statistics—Cause 1981. England and Wales. Series GH2, No. 8. HMSO, London (1983).

Nilsson, M.-I., Meresaar, U., and Anggard, E. (1982). Clinical pharmacokinetics of methadone. *Acta anaesth. Scand.* **26,** Suppl. 74, 66.

Twycross, R. G. (1978). Relief of pain. In *The management of terminal disease* (ed. C. Saunders) p. 65. Edward Arnold, London.

Vanderpool, H. Y. (1978). The ethics of terminal care. *J. Am. med. Ass.* **239,** 850.

Verebely, K., Volavka, J., Mule, S., and Resnick, R. (1975). Methadone in man: pharma-cokinetic and excretion studies in acute and chronic treatment. *Clin. Pharmacol. Ther.* **18,** 180.

Welsh, J., Stuart, J. F. B., Habeshaw, T., Blackie, R., Whitehill, D., Setanoians, A., Milstead, R. A. V., and Calman, K. C. (1983). A comparative pharmacokinetic study of morphine sulphate solution and MST Continus 30 mg tablets in conditions expected to allow steady-state drug levels. In *Methods of morphine estimation in biological fluids and the concept of free morphine* (ed. J. F. B. Stuart). Royal Society of Medicine International Congress and Symposium Series, No. 58, p. 9. Royal Society of Medicine/Academic Press, London.

Controlled-release morphine in advanced cancer pain

C. B. REGNARD and F. RANDELL

Macmillan Continuing Care Unit,
Christchurch Hospital,
Christchurch,
Dorset

Introduction

The four-hourly administration of simple morphine or diamorphine solution remains an effective choice in controlling the pain of advanced cancer. However, the development of controlled-release morphine sulphate (MST Continus tablets, Napp Laboratories Ltd.), in tablet form and with an 8–12-hourly dosage regimen offers practical advantages.

Initially we administer four-hourly diamorphine solution orally since the dose can be titrated upwards within days until a patient is pain-free. It is then our usual practice to cross patients over to controlled-release morphine sulphate tablets when this is practicable. We report on an evaluation of this practice.

Methods

All patients gave full, informed consent and patients who were too ill or simply too tired to be evaluated were not disturbed. Pain, drowsiness, and nausea were assessed by conventional, uniform, visual analogue scales (VAS). Pain scores were also derived from the McGill pain questionnaire (MPQ), administered as described by Melzack (1975). VAS were completed by patients daily for one week, then weekly for two months. MPQ scores were obtained on the last day on diamorphine and one week after commencing controlled-release morphine. Fifteen potential opioid side-effects were assessed by patients on a four-point scale (absent, mild, moderate, severe), at the same time as the MPQ, and also on the first day on controlled-release morphine: drowsiness, nausea, vomiting, constipation, sweating, flushing, itching, palpitations, nightmares, confusion, lethargy, dry mouth, anorexia, and feelings of unreality.

Advances in Morphine Therapy. The 1983 International Symposium on Pain Control, edited by E. Wilkes, 1984: Royal Society of Medicine International Congress and Symposium Series No. 64, published by the Royal Society of Medicine.

Results

Forty-three patients were accepted but 13 became too ill to continue. A further five patients were excluded because of new sites of pain or a poor response to diamorphine (shown by a reduction in VAS or MPQ scores of less than 50 per cent compared to the original severity of their pain). One patient refused to cross over and another was unable to swallow the controlled-release morphine sulphate tablets. The remaining 23 patients had a mean age of 65 years and their cancers had been diagnosed a median time of 40 months before evaluation.

On changing from diamorphine to controlled-release morphine sulphate a 50 per cent increase in the 24-hour dose was made initially because of established potency differences between these two opioids (Twycross 1977, 1981). It became clear that the first 10 patients at this ratio (1 : 1.5) were suffering increased side-effects on changing to controlled-release morphine sulphate. The remaining 13 patients were therefore continued at a diamorphine to controlled-release morphine ratio of 1 : 1.

There was little change in pain VAS scores on crossing over to controlled-release morphine sulphate (Fig. 1) and no significant difference at either ratio on testing with the Wilcoxan signed-rank test. Mean MPQ scores after one week on controlled-release morphine also showed no significant change on rank testing at either ratio.

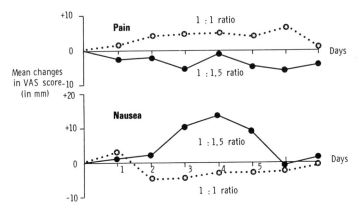

Fig. 1. Mean changes in visual analogue scale (VAS) scores for pain and nausea during the first week on controlled-release morphine sulphate tablets, and following a crossover from oral diamorphine at either a 1 : 1.5 or a 1 : 1 ratio.

Mean nausea VAS scores increased at four days at the 1 : 1.5 ratio (Fig. 1). After one week on controlled-release morphine sulphate patients at the 1 : 1.5 ratio had reported 25 increases on the four-point scale for potential opioid side-effects, compared to 18 decreases (Table 1). However, at the 1 : 1 ratio there were nine increases and 34 decreases in severity (Table 2).

Conclusions

Four-hourly controlled-release morphine sulphate tablets appear as effective in relieving cancer pain as diamorphine hydrochloride solution. The usual practice of increasing 24-hour doses by 50 per cent when changing from oral diamorphine to

Table 1

Changes in severity of opiate side-effects
(first day on MST Continus tablets)

Side-effect	1 : 1.5	1 : 1
Drowsiness	+5	−1
Vomiting	+4	+2
Nausea	+3	−1
Confusion	+4	0
Dizziness	+4	−1
Feelings of unreality	+3	0
Lethargy	+2	−1
Dry mouth	+1	+2
Nightmares	+1	0
Itching	0	0
Anorexia	0	+2
Flushing	−1	0
Constipation	−2	+1
Palpitations	−1	0
Sweating	−4	−1
	+19	**+2**
	(−14 +33)	(−12 +14)

Table 2

Changes in severity of opiate side-effects
(after one week on MST Continus tablets)

Side-effect	1 : 1.5	1 : 1
Drowsiness	+2	−5
Vomiting	+3	0
Nausea	−1	−2
Confusion	+1	0
Dizziness	+1	−1
Feelings of unreality	+1	−3
Lethargy	−1	−3
Dry mouth	+2	−1
Nightmares	+2	−2
Itching	0	−1
Anorexia	+5	−1
Flushing	0	−1
Constipation	−5	−1
Palpitations	0	0
Sweating	−3	−4
	+7	**−25**
	(−18 +25)	(−34 +9)

morphine increases side-effects if controlled-release morphine sulphate is used. A pharmacokinetic study (Welsh *et al*. 1983) has confirmed that controlled-release morphine sulphate produces higher and more prolonged plasma levels than oral morphine sulphate solution, even though the 24-hour dose of morphine solution was 50 per cent greater. Since the potency ratio of oral morphine solution to oral diamorphine solution is 1 : 1.5 (Twycross 1981), one would expect the same 24-hour doses of oral diamorphine solution and controlled-release tablets to be equianalgesic. Our preliminary evaluation suggests this supposition is correct, and this now needs to be confirmed by a larger-scale, double-blind, crossover trial.

Acknowledgements

We thank Napp Laboratories Ltd. for their help in this evaluation.

References

Melzack, R. (1975). The McGill pain questionnaire: major properties and scoring methods. *Pain* **1,** 277.
Twycross, R. G. (1977). Choice of strong analgesic in terminal cancer: diamorphine or morphine? *Pain* **3,** 93.
—— (1981). Controlled-release morphine tablets. (Letter.) *Lancet* **i,** 892.
Welsh, J. Stuart, J. F. B., Habeshaw, T., Blackie, K., Whitehill, D., Setanoians, A., Milstead, R. A. V., and Calman, K. C. (1983). A comparative pharmacokinetic study of morphine sulphate solution and MST Continus 30 mg tablets in conditions expected to allow steady state drug levels. In *Methods of morphine estimation in biological fluids and the concept of free morphine* (ed. J. F. B. Stuart). Royal Society of Medicine International Congress Symposium Series No. 58, p. 9. Royal Society of Medicine/Academic Press, London.

Epidural morphine in the home treatment of cancer pain

M. S. CHAYEN

*Khilat Padua 12,
Tel Aviv,
Israel*

Introduction

Severe intractable pain from terminal disease is often difficult to treat. The classic method is to use morphine or diamorphine administered by mouth or by intramuscular injection. Advancing technology and expertise has opened up a new route, however.

The epidural route for the administration of anaesthetic agents is increasing in popularity especially in obstetrics. It is logical, therefore, if one wishes to relieve central pain, to administer an opiate epidurally. This ensures that the opiate reaches the required site of action and that less opiate needs to be used.

We report here our experience of the administration of epidural morphine in 40 patients suffering from severe pain of malignant origin.

Method

An epidural catheter with a 2 μm filter was inserted aseptically either at the 2nd–4th lumbar region or mid-thorax. The catheter was then secured to the chest. The initial dose of morphine was administered by the physician with subsequent doses given by a nurse, relative, or even the patient himself. The dose of morphine sulphate used was 2 mg in 10 ml of sterile saline.

Precautions

Whilst in the study, as well as routinely, patients are kept under observation during the day of the initial injection. After stabilization they are sent home and receive daily

Advances in Morphine Therapy. The 1983 International Symposium on Pain Control, edited by E. Wilkes, 1984: Royal Society of Medicine International Congress and Symposium Series No. 64, published by the Royal Society of Medicine.

visits by the home care unit. They record their temperature nightly with instructions to report any rise above 30 °C or any local inflammation occurring at the site of the insertion of the catheter. Occasionally the catheter needs to be changed if (i) it slipped out of place, or (ii) in some cases (after irradiation of the block) the patient refused the change and as long as six weeks has elapsed with the same catheter in place.

Results

Thirty-eight out of the 40 patients obtained good relief by the use of epidural morphine. Pain relief normally occurred 12–20 minutes after the injection of 2 mg in 10 ml saline. The two other cases that failed to achieve pain relief had heavy visceral involvement by the tumour. Pain relief varied in length from as little as one day to five months.

Morphine tolerance

Morphine tolerance developed in five patients after five days' treatment. They therefore received 10 ml of 1 per cent lidocaine via the epidural catheter and were then able to resume their morphine therapy. This treatment was thereafter successfully repeated as the patient became tolerant to morphine again. We are unable to explain this phenomenon.

Complications and side-effects

These are summarized in Table 1.

Table 1
Complications and side-effects

Changes in blood pressure or pulse rate	None
Urinary retention	None
Itching	1 (did not recur)
Delayed respiratory depression	None
Local infection	1 mild in skin 1 growth of pyocyaneus obtained from the tip of the catheter. The patient was symptomless and this may have been an accidental contamination
Neurological (impairment of motor function, positional sense, loss of identification of pin prick, heat or cold)	None
Drowsiness	None

Conclusions

Morphine given via the epidural route is an alternative route of administration with a low incidence of side-effects. It is, however, a rather cumbersome method and may only be useful in a limited number of patients. The action and interaction of the lidocaine on the morphine receptors is, however, of great interest and warrants further investigation.

High systemic relative bioavailability of oral morphine in both solution and sustained-release formulation

H. J. McQUAY, R. A. MOORE, R. E. S. BULLINGHAM, DAWN CARROLL,
D. BALDWIN, M. C. ALLEN, C. J. GLYNN, and J. W. LLOYD

*Oxford Regional Pain Relief Unit, Abingdon,
and Nuffield Departments of Anaesthetics and Clinical Biochemistry,
Radcliffe Infirmary,
Oxford*

Summary

In a within-patient crossover study on five patients requiring oral narcotic therapy for the treatment of chronic pain, plasma morphine concentrations were compared for 24 hours after 10 mg intravenous morphine sulphate, 10 mg morphine sulphate solution [MSS] and 10 mg MST Continus tablets. The plasma levels between 30 and 120 minutes were significantly higher after MSS than after MST. Between 300 minutes and 24 hours the plasma morphine concentrations after MST were significantly higher than after MSS. The systemic clearance of morphine over the 24-hour study period was significantly lower after MST, and the relative availability was significantly higher. The relative availability for both oral formulations was about 100 per cent higher than previously estimated.

Introduction

Oral morphine is an established method of treating severe chronic pain because the oral route can give as good relief as parenteral doses, and the advantage of the parenteral routes is limited to those circumstances where oral doses are impracticable or rapid pain relief is required.

Oral morphine is commonly given as a liquid preparation, at four-hourly intervals. A 'slow-release' formulation which reduced the number of daily doses required could be of benefit to the patients, provided that its release was neither too slow nor incomplete. This study was designed to compare the plasma morphine concentrations

Advances in Morphine Therapy. The 1983 International Symposium on Pain Control, edited by E. Wilkes, 1984: Royal Society of Medicine International Congress and Symposium Series No. 64, published by the Royal Society of Medicine.

after oral morphine solution with those from a commercially available sustained-release formulation. Such kinetic comparison is important for clinical use of novel formulations and to the design of studies comparing the effect of standard and novel preparations.

Methods

Five patients who required oral narcotic therapy were selected from those attending the Oxford Regional Pain Relief Unit. They were aged between 41 and 79 years (63.2 ± 7, mean $\pm$ SEM), weighed 68 to 80 kg (73 ± 2) and there were four females and one male. None suffered from clinically apparent hepatic, renal, cardiac, respiratory or psychiatric disorder, or took drugs known to interfere with the morphine assay. The study was approved by the hospital ethics committee and informed consent was obtained from the patients.

The study design was open and within patient crossover. Each patient received an intravenous (i.v.) dose of morphine sulphate pentahydrate 10 mg (26.4 μmol morphine sulphate injection BP, Evans Medical, Greenford, Middlesex) on the first study day. On a second day they were given 10 mg of morphine sulphate pentahydrate as an oral slow-release morphine [MST] (MST Continus tablets, Napp Laboratories Ltd.), with 100 ml of tap water, and on a third day they received oral morphine solution 10 mg [MSS] (morphine sulphate injection BP drawn up in via syringe and needle, injected into 50 ml of tap water which the patient drank, followed immediately by a further 50 ml of tap water. The ampoules were not rinsed out). Studies were run on consecutive days when possible; one patient (7) had MSS before MST.

Intravenous injection of 10 mg morphine sulphate diluted to 20 ml with 0.9 per cent w/v normal saline was given over one minute into an i.v. line in the arm. Venous samples (time from the end of injection) were taken from the contralateral arm pre-injection and at 1, 2, 5, 7.5, 10, 20, 30, 40, 60, 90, 120, 150, 180, 210, 240, 300, 360, 720, and 1440 minutes. Sample timing for the oral doses was pretreatment (0), 30, 60, 90, 120, 150, 180, 210, 240, 300, 360, 720, and 1440 minutes. Samples were taken into lithium heparin tubes, separated within one hour and stored frozen until analysis.

Patients were kept supine for at least one hour after the test dose and then allowed up at the discretion of the nurse. They had a light breakfast on the day of study before the dose and tea and toast were given if needed between the first and sixth hours; thereafter patients ate normally.

Plasma morphine concentrations were determined by radioimmunoassay using ^{125}I-labelled morphine prepared in the Nuffield Department of Clinical Biochemistry with a specific antiserum exhibiting < 1 per cent cross-reactivity with either morphine-3-glucuronide or normorphine (Moore et al. 1984a). The method has been validated using high-pressure liquid chromatography with electrochemical detection (Moore et al. 1984b). Time to maximum plasma concentration (t_{max}), peak plasma concentration (Cp_{max}), time when plasma morphine concentration rose above 100 nmol/l ($t > 100$) and time when plasma morphine concentration fell below 100 nmol/l ($t < 100$) were determined from individual patient plasma morphine concentration data. An area under the curve to 24 hours ($AUC_{24\,h}$) of plasma morphine concentration against time was obtained using a trapezoidal rule. Systemic clearance over 24 hours ($Cl_{s24\,h}$) was obtained for each patient by dividing the dose by the $AUC_{24\,h}$. Relative bioavailability of the oral formulations was calculated by dividing the $AUC_{24\,h}$ of the oral doses by the $AUC_{24\,h}$ of the intravenous dose. The conversion factor for SI units (nmol/l) to ng/ml morphine base was 1/2.64.

The paired 't' test was used to test for significance of differences; the level of significance was taken as $p < 0.05$.

Results

Mean plasma morphine concentrations following the different oral morphine formulations are shown in Table 1. The mean baseline plasma morphine concentrations for MSS and MST were not the same as the 1440 minute values for the preceding dose because the studies did not always follow on consecutive days.

Table 1
Plasma morphine concentrations (nmol/1, mean ± SEM)

Time (min)	i.v. morphine sulphate ($n = 5$)	Oral morphine sulphate solution ($n = 5$)	Oral MST Continus ($n = 5$)	p
0	0	15 ± 10	23 ± 8	NS
30	324 ± 64	125 ± 24	30 ± 9	0.01
60	323 ± 55	213 ± 55	64 ± 18	0.01
90	291 ± 58	222 ± 52	79 ± 15	0.01
120	242 ± 46	212 ± 32	127 ± 19	0.01
150	210 ± 55*	187 ± 18	155 ± 16	NS
180	242 ± 46	178 ± 18	165 ± 19	NS
210	191 ± 48*	149 ± 18	179 ± 25	NS
240	166 ± 44	137 ± 18	182 ± 26	NS
300	142 ± 38	118 ± 18	180 ± 25	0.01
360	122 ± 36	103 ± 17	190 ± 31*	0.01
720	51 ± 20	57 ± 14	79 ± 17	0.01
1440	36 ± 7	31 ± 5	45 ± 8	NS

Significance from paired 't' test.
* $N = 4$.

The baseline plasma morphine concentrations for MSS and MST compared within-patient were not significantly different (paired 't' test). By 30 minutes, the plasma morphine concentrations after MSS were significantly higher than after MST (Table 1 and Fig. 1). This significant difference was maintained up to and including the 120 minute sample. There was no significant difference at 150, 180, 210 or 240 minutes, but from 300 to 1440 minutes the plasma morphine concentrations were significantly higher for MST than for MSS.

The t_{max} was significantly delayed by about 130 minutes on average after MST compared with MSS but there was no significant difference in Cp_{max}. The time by which a concentration of > 100 nmol/l ($t > 100$) was reached was significantly shorter with MSS (54 ± 18 min, mean ± SEM) than with MST (114 ± 15 min). The time by which a concentration of less than 100 nmol/l ($t < 100$) was regained was significantly shorter with MSS (348 ± 98 min) than with MST (432 ± 72 min). There was no significant difference in the time (about 300 minutes) over which a plasma morphine concentration of greater than 100 nmol/l was sustained.

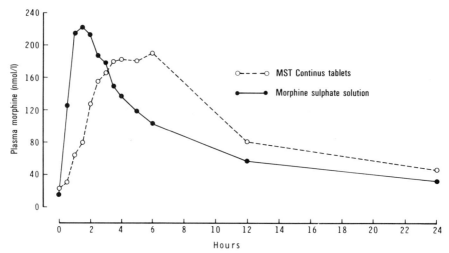

Fig. 1. *Plasma morphine concentration (nmol/l) of morphine sulphate solution 10 mg and MST Continus tablets 10 mg.*

While there was no significant difference in the $AUC_{24 h}$ between the i.v. dose and either MSS or MST, there was a significantly greater $AUC_{24 h}$ after MST compared with MSS on the paired 't' test. The mean ratio of $AUC_{24 h}$ MST to $AUC_{24 h}$ MSS was 1.2 ± 0.03 (SEM, range 1.1–1.25). Similarly, with no difference in $AUC_{24 h}$ between the i.v. dose and either oral formulation, the $Cl_{s24 h}$ was significantly lower after MST compared with MSS. The relative availability of the MST dose (mean 122 per cent) was significantly greater than that of MSS (mean 100 per cent).

Discussion

These results showed that the absorption of morphine from oral MST was delayed by about two hours in comparison with oral MSS, although peak plasma concentrations were not significantly different. The significantly greater $AUC_{24 h}$ with MST reflected the significantly higher plasma morphine concentrations from five to 24 hours; the lower $Cl_{s24 h}$ and greater relative availability derived from the $AUC_{24 h}$ were also significantly different from MSS, but not from the i.v. dose.

While the experimental design, with doses given on successive days, necessarily leads to an order effect such that the preceding dose makes a contribution to the AUC of the succeeding dose, this contribution does not affect the conclusions, first because there was no significant difference within the patients between the plasma morphine concentrations at the start of the MST and MSS studies, and second because such an order effect should have increased the $AUC_{24 h}$ from the MSS, which was given third, relatively more than for MST, which was given second. In all five patients the $AUC_{24 h}$ for MST was greater than for MSS.

The relative availabilities for both oral dose were higher than expected in view of the calculated extraction ratio for morphine of 0.7 (Stanski *et al.* 1978). The validity of such an extraction ratio, however, rests on the premise that morphine plasma clearance is relatively high, approximatly 14 ml/min/kg compared with a hepatic blood flow of 21 ml/min/kg.

The plasma clearance of morphine is subject to wide variation; mean published values range from 5 to 28 ml/min/kg with a range for individual subjects of 2 to 40 ml/min/kg. A similar variation has been noted for fentanyl (Mather 1983). This phenomenon is not related to the type of assay because it has been found with different assay systems and because the same investigators using the same assay system have obtained both high and low mean clearance data. If the lowest figure for morphine plasma clearance is correct, then the hepatic extraction ratio will be much less than 0.7, and the relative oral availability much higher than 30 per cent.

Rather than calculate the extraction ratio, plasma morphine concentrations after oral and intravenous doses may be compared in the same patient, and this approach was taken in the present study. Previous work (Sawe *et al.* 1981) with low i.v. doses and oral doses of 20–30 mg morphine showed oral availability to be as high as 64 per cent. In the present study, using 10 mg i.v. and 10 mg orally, it was approximately 100 per cent for both MSS and MST. Such a high availability for oral morphine may be explained by predominantly renal rather than hepatic morphine metabolism within the plasma morphine concentration range studied (see chapter by McQuay *et al.*, pp. 111–22).

The data also supported MST as being a sustained release preparation. First the plasma morphine concentrations after MST were the same or significantly greater than those from MSS from 2.5 to 24 hours after the dose. Secondly, the peak plasma morphine concentration after MST was about four hours and the mean plasma concentration after six hours was still 190 nmol/l. Although the interval during which plasma morphine concentrations were greater than 100 nmol/l was not greater for MST than for MSS, this was an artefactual result because there were only two sample times after the six-hour sample.

The clinical implications of the current study for single dose use of MST are that a loading dose parenterally or as premedicant may be necessary to get round the slower onset time of MST compared with MSS. Slow onset may explain the relative failure of MST in the acute setting when rapid analgesia was required (Hanks *et al.* 1981). For multiple dose use a lower number of daily doses of MST should produce plasma morphine concentrations equivalent to those seen with four- or six-hourly MSS dosing. As yet there is no controlled effect data to substantiate this.

Acknowledgements

We would like to thank the patients of the Oxford Regional Pain Relief Unit for taking part in the study, and the staff for all their help. DC was supported by the Cancer Research Campaign; financial support was also received from the Medical Research Council and Oxford Regional Health Authority.

References

Hanks, G. W., Rose, N. M., Aherne, G. W., and Piall, E. M. (1981). Analgesic effect of morphine tablets. *Lancet* **i,** 732.

Mather, L. E. (1983). Clinical pharmacokinetics of fentanyl and its newer derivatives. *Clin. Pharmacokinet.* **8,** 422.

Moore, R. A., Baldwin, D., Allen, M. C., Watson, P. J. Q., Bullingham, R. E. S., and McQuay, H. J. (1984*a*). Sensitive and specific morphine radioimmunoassay with iodine label: pharmacokinetics of morphine in man after intravenous administration. *Annls clin. Biochem.*, in press.

—— McQuay, H. J., and Bullingham, R. E. S. (1984*b*). HPLC of morphine with electrochemical detection: analysis in human plasma. *Annls clin. Biochem.*, in press.

Sawe, J., Dahlstrom, B., Paalzow, L., and Rane, A. (1981). Morphine kinetics in cancer patients. *Clin. Pharmacol. Ther.* **30,** 629.

Stanski, D. R., Greenblatt, D. J., and Lowenstein, E. (1978). Kinetics of intravenous and intramuscular morphine. *Clin. Pharmacol. Ther.* **24,** 52.

Session 3: Morphine: 200 years on
What have we learnt?

Introduction

A. DOENICKE

*Chirug. Univ. Klinik. u. Poliklinik,
Munchen–Innenstadt,
Munchen*

Despite the rapid development of anaesthesiology over the last 30 years with, for example, the introduction of powerful inhalation anaesthetics (halothane, enflurane), anaesthetists are constantly reminded of the discovery of morphine by Sertürner. Potentiated anesthesia during the years 1952–1956, neuroleptanalgesia from 1959 onwards, intrathecal administration of morphine for combatting postoperative pain, and also the treatment of severe tumour pain would have been inconceivable without analgesic components of the morphine type. The use of morphine anaesthesia has grown in the USA over the last 10 years. Morphine is still preferred by many anaesthetists as a premedication. It was therefore appropriate that in June of this year we anaesthetists should have marked the 200th anniversary of the pharmacist's birth with an international symposium on the subject of pain, its research and treatment, at Göttingen and Einbeck.

Friedrich Wilhelm Adam Sertürner was born in Neuhaus, near Paderborn, on 19 June 1783. His life falls broadly into three main periods:

1. Childhood and pharmacist's apprenticeship in Paderborn; at the age of 21, while a pharmacist's assistant at the court pharmacy, he discovered in poppy juice a base, which he called morphium. He made this knowledge public by means of a number of letters in Trommsdorff's *Journal der Pharmacie* in 1805 and 1806.

2. Two and a half years after finishing his apprenticeship, he moved to Einbeck and became an assistant at the town hall pharmacy in 1806. He set up his own business there in 1809.

He completed his studies on morphium and presented his findings to the public—and therefore to criticism—with a paper in the *Annalen der Physik* 1817. His first revelations, which had been published as letters in 1805, had attracted little attention.

Even while proof-reading this paper, Sertürner was able to add new knowledge about morphium's crystals in an appendix and to define the morphine crystal of Derosne's opium salt and that of meconic acid.

Before Sertürner investigated the effects of morphium on the human body, he observed what happened when a dog was given this substance. 'After administering the substance, sleep set in immediately and later vomiting. On renewed intake, everything was vomited up, but the inclination to sleep persisted for several hours.'

Advances in Morphine Therapy. The 1983 International Symposium on Pain Control, edited by E. Wilkes, 1984: Royal Society of Medicine International Congress and Symposium Series No. 64, published by the Royal Society of Medicine.

The step from preclinical to clinical experiment gives rise to problems with every new substance. The experiment on three people, none of whom was more than 17 years old, who together with Sertürner took morphine, consequently took a dramatic course. 'I gave each person only $\frac{1}{2}$ grain dissolved in $\frac{1}{2}$ dram alcohol and diluted with a few ounces of water. A general redness, which was even visible in the eyes, spread over the face, especially the cheeks, and life activity appeared to be generally heightened. When after $\frac{1}{2}$ hour another $\frac{1}{2}$ grain of morphium was taken, this condition increased noticeably, with a transitory inclination to vomit and a dull pain in the head with stupor. Without waiting for the results, which would perhaps already have been very bad, we took another $\frac{1}{2}$ grain of morphium $\frac{1}{4}$ hour later in the form of undissolved coarse powder, with 10 drops of alcohol and $\frac{1}{2}$ ounce of water. The result was rapid in the 3 young men and extremely distinct. There was pain in the stomach, exhaustion and severe stupor bordering on unconsciousness. I too had the same fate; as I lay, I entered a dream-like state, and could feel a slight twitching in the extremities and in particular the arms, and this as it were accompanied the pulse.'

Sertürner and his three young test subjects had taken almost 1/10 gram of morphine, precisely three times the dose considered today to be the maximum.

'Lack of bowel opening and appetite, stupor, pain in the head and body disappeared only after a few days. Judging by my own highly unpleasant experience, morphium acts as a violent poison even in small doses.' Despite his description of these side-effects. Sertürner also indicated that therapeutic effects in illness could probably be expected from the various morphine salts, e.g. violent toothache which would not abate after taking opium might be relieved by a solution of morphium in alcohol.

Using precise methods of investigation, the Boston study group of Philbin, Moss, and Savarese were able to prove in 1982 that morphine releases histamine in man under clinical conditions. Their results also pointed out that fentanyl—a modern morphine derivative—does not release any histamine. Furthermore, they succeeded in preventing the histamine-dependent cardiac circulatory effects with H_1 and H_2 receptor antagonists.

In contrast to our Bostonian friends, our study group (Doenicke, Lorenz) indicated at the 5th Sertürner Workshop in Einbeck that: 'very small amounts of fentanyl such as are used for premedication are capable of releasing histamine.' However, since this investigation was only carried out on a small number of test subjects and so does not hold out against scientific statistical criteria, we decided in February/March 1983 to test fentanyl and alfentanil on 32 patients in a randomized prospective study. Here too, our aim was to prove that these modern analgesics can release histamine in some cases. However, the clinical symptoms were considerably more interesting. The side-effects observed by Sertürner 180 years ago also occurred with fentanyl/alfentanil. Today, we refer to these cutaneous reactions as cutaneous anaphylaxis if the histamine in plasma does not rise above 1 ng/ml.

The symptoms observed seldom go together with a systemic reaction, i.e. hypotension. They are in fact the consequence of increased histamine release (more than 1 ng/ml). The redness with formation of weals occurred as described by Sertürner, mainly on the face and the upper half of the body.

Let us return to Sertürner's decisive publications between 1805 and 1817, in which he recognized morphium as 'a soporific and analgesic principle' in opium and furnished proof of its alkaline character. With this publication he became the discoverer of a new class of plant substances—the alkaloids.

After 1817, an intensive search for further similar substances began worldwide.

Morphine and quinine were already listed in the Hamburg pharmacopoeia of 1842, and cinchonine and strychnine were added in 1827.

3. In the third stage of his life from 1820 onwards, Sertürner hoped to find quieter circumstances in Hamlin, where he took over the town hall pharmacy. A happy family life made it possible for Sertürner to pursue his scientific inclinations.

Yet he believed that he had taken on a great responsibility with the discovery of morphium, and this weighed heavily on him. In addition, the consequences of the experiments he had carried out on himself became apparent with advancing age; morphium did not pass him by without a trace either.

At the age of 58, Friedrich Wilhelm Adam Sertürner died in Hamlin; he was buried in the small chapel of St. Bartholomew (first half of the fifteenth century) before the gates of Einbeck.

In retrospect, the consequences of Sertürner's discovery and with them his importance for posterity can be summed up as follows: with the foundation of alkaloid chemistry, doctors could for the first time measure out precisely, and in a clearly defined composition, plant medicines which had been in use since time immemorial, and this enabled their effect to be calculated. The isolation of morphine enabled doctors to treat successfully very severe pain states.

How great a blessing morphine has become for the physician despite the dangers of habituation emerges from the statement made by the director of the Münster University Hospital, Paul Krause, who wrote in 1925: 'Without morphium I would not want to be a doctor. In the hands of the experienced doctor it is the friend which takes away the pain.'

Although a succession of morphine-like substances have been manufactured synthetically over the last 50 years, morphine is still as indispensable as ever for the relief of very severe pain.

The year 1983, the 200th anniversary of Friedrich Wilhelm Sertürner's birth, not only brought with it anniversary celebrations in Paderborn and Einbeck, but also forced us to define our position at the international Sertürner Symposium in Göttingen. Scientifically speaking, we now know a considerable amount about the phenomenon of pain, but the reality is that the patient tormented by cancer pain is often left to his own devices.

'Human death should mean a dignified death, but who can uphold dignity while writhing in pain?' (Paul Lüth).

There are no out-patient or in-patient pain clinics in the municipal or state hospitals. If such institutions are available it is only thanks to the private initiative of interested doctors who help the sufferer in their spare time.

Additional house-officer posts have as yet not been authorized by the state (at least this is the case in Bavaria).

Thanks to cancer aid, 30 million DM are available for cancer prevention, but for cancer pain—the pain before death—there is no money at all.

So the awkward realization remains that today not only medicine, but also state authorities have been unforthcoming where pain is concerned.

World Health Organization cancer pain-relief programme

V. VENTAFRIDDA and M. SWERDLOW

Division of Pain Therapy,
Istituto Nazionali Tumori,
Milan,
and Cancer Pain Relief Programme,
World Health Organization,
Geneva

Almost all the data we have on the incidence of cancer pain is derived from investigations carried out in hospitals, hospices or urban studies in western countries, particularly in the United Kingdom and the United States of America and most of the patients were at a pre-terminal or terminal stage. It is clear from these data that even in these 'medically affluent' areas, a significant proportion of patients are not given adequate relief of pain, despite the fact that a high degree of expertise in the treatment of intractable pain now exists.

If there are such deficiencies in the management of cancer pain in the developed countries, what about the rest of the world where recent advances in pain therapy are now only just starting to be introduced into teaching hospitals? Traditional and tribal methods (be it herbs, spells or acupuncture) may be widely used and can indeed be efficacious, although no data are available at present. However, conversations with third-world representatives and personal observations suggest that for much of the world, most of the population, especially the rural dwellers, are offered little or nothing at all in the way of effective pain relief.

In the third world there are many basic difficulties and problems. In many developing countries 60–80 per cent of the population do not have constant access even to essential drugs; hospitals in the towns and cities tend to get priority in drug allocation to the detriment of people living in rural areas.

In most developing countries cancer patients arrive at treatment centres (if at all) with advanced disease at a stage too late for meaningful treatment. Rather than offering marginally efficient and highly expensive therapy, often with high morbidity, would it not be better to offer these incurable cancer patients efficient pain relief so that they die without unnecessary suffering? Incurable patients could then be with their family and friends during their final weeks. There are 45–50 million deaths per year of whom at a conservative estimate 10 per cent are due to cancer and if half of

Advances in Morphine Therapy. The 1983 International Symposium on Pain Control, edited by E. Wilkes, 1984: Royal Society of Medicine International Congress and Symposium Series No. 64, published by the Royal Society of Medicine.

these have pain at some stage of the disease, one sees that the number involved is truly enormous.

In 1981 the World Health Organization commenced a long-term programme aimed at global provision of basic cancer pain relief. The first phase of this programme was carried out in a number of countries and comprised a study of the present incidence of cancer pain, methods being used for relief and the effectiveness of those methods. For this purpose questionnaires were completed at single interviews with 250 successive out-patients following clinical diagnosis of cancer.

The next phase was to produce a practical handbook of cancer pain relief therapy. This was prepared at a consultation which was held in Milan in October 1982. Six international experts in the treatment of pain discussed in depth and evolved a handbook on cancer pain and its management. Obviously the only universally applicable means of providing relief is pharmacological; however, the approach is comprehensive including radiotherapy, oncology, and total care.

The first section of the handbook explains the causes of pain in cancer patients and emphasizes the need to assess the types of pain in order to determine the appropriate drug therapy. The various drugs which are advocated for analgesia are described in detail including their pharmacodynamics and side-effects. The approach to the management of medication is followed step by step—proceeding from initial non-narcotic drugs via weak narcotics to strong narcotics. In addition the handbook gives the indications for the use of adjuvant drugs such as psychotropics, anticonvulsants, antiemetics, and steroids. A section is included on the factors affecting choice of drug and dosage such as liver and kidney impairment, tropical diseases, and malnutrition.

The goal of these guidelines is to provide a clear plan of action for health-care personnel. The handbook will be available to doctors throughout the world but it is particularly intended for the doctor working in the more peripheral parts of the under-developed countries who have at present very little access to information. The guidelines are intended for general adaptation to conditions in different countries and communities and will be modified locally to suit the users.

The 'field-testing' of the draft guidelines is now being set up and this testing is expected to take about three years. Initially the help of major cancer centres will be enlisted in developed and developing countries and later testing will be done in a number of regional health care centres. The studies will include both the feasibility of clinical implementation of the guidlines as well as such aspects as drug availability, storage, and legal controls. For some studies the population will be re-surveyed after a specific interval to determine the effectiveness and safety of the cancer pain therapies administered.

Some of the ideal characteristics of drugs to be included would be low cost without compromise on quality, lack of need for refrigeration, storage and stability under wide variations in climate and convenience of administration in simple surroundings. The problem of availability, legislation and registration of potent drugs will need solution.

The next step will be the identification of a steering committee to provide expert guidance to the progamme and the institution of a World Health Organization Collaborating Centre at the Division of Pain Therapy, National Cancer Institute of Milan, Italy, to co-ordinate the necessary field research and evaluation. A central office will be set up to be responsible for collecting and synthesizing available global information relating to cancer pain therapy including information on the distribution, legislation and registration of the major analgesics. This office will disseminate the information by periodic reports.

Target regions are being identified in specific developed and developing countries which have the necessary infrastructure for conducting a population-based study of the incidence and prevalence of cancer pain and the appropriate epidemiological studies will be conducted.

In 1986 it is planned that the World Health Organization will call an Expert Meeting to consider all available information including the data resulting from the field testing, in order to decide which drugs and preparations and dosages should be recommended. The guideline handbook will then be revised to form the basis of the definitive World Health Organization Cancer Pain Relief Programme and will be universally promoted, especially via national cancer programmes and policies. They will also decide on the logistical and legal processes which will be needed to implement globally the expert recommendations. The recommended approaches, including the availability of drugs will then be promoted as part of national health policies in member states.

Obviously a widespread educational programme will have to accompany the introduction of the recommended therapy. The educational process will commence with the medical and nursing staff of hospitals and will then be extended to health-centre staff and health workers in villages and more remote communities. The treatment will have to be acceptable and accessible to the people.

Finally, the global implementation of the programme will be effected in 1986-90. Basic educational materials, press releases, and training courses suitable for various audiences (medical, legislators, administrators, etc.) will be developed. These materials will be modified at a local level as necessary. Cancer physician awareness of the programme will also be promoted by international meetings and publications.

We believe that if the drugs and knowledge which already exist were properly applied universally then we could eliminate much of the pain at present suffered by cancer patients. Cancer pain relief should become the right of every cancer sufferer within the reach of primary health care services.

The 1983 International Symposium on Pain Control

Summary of the symposium and closing remarks

E. WILKES

We have had, I think, a most interesting and valuable few days. We started off with a comprehensive overview of pain systems from Professor Illia Jurna in all the areas involved with injury and pain. He reminded us of the importance of prostaglandin E_2 and that morphine reduces or slows conduction in peripheral nerve fibres. Professor Graham Smith described (and this does not happen only in postoperative analgesia) how senior doctors delegate to junior doctors who delegate to poorly educated nurses. I also accept the whole problem which other speakers and other chairmen have mentioned about doctor–nurse relationships and how, when these relationships are impaired, it is the patient who pays the price. I accept at once that to some senior nursing colleagues it may be that the nursing process is merely a handy weapon in the perpetual guerilla war being waged between doctor and senior nurse, especially across the Atlantic. I think, however, it is necessary to say that so far as my own lengthy, but anecdotal experience is concerned, I am hearing a great deal more criticism from nurses about the analgesic regimens of the doctors.

It is extremely important that analgesia be seen as an interdisciplinary responsibility. Doctor and nurse are either one, or they are failures in their professional responsibilities.

This leads me to another point, which, of course, I do not need to say to such a lively and imaginative audience. Pain control in the home, in out-patients, among the family doctors, among the 'anguished in spirit'; these must be interdisciplinary responsibilities. The pain clinic and hospice unit must have more skills than any one person may be able to handle.

We did have a written question, which we did not have time to touch on, which queried the dedication—if that is the right word—of so many hospice teams to the opiates, to the exclusion of other more specific techniques. I think that it is very easy to produce—in Professor Baum's phrase—'a false confrontation' with, on the one hand, the stereotype of the slashing, needle-hungry anaesthetist and on the other, the hospice

Advances in Morphine Therapy. The 1983 International Symposium on Pain Control, edited by E. Wilkes, 1984: Royal Society of Medicine International Congress and Symposium Series No. 64, published by the Royal Society of Medicine.

medical director who is very happy when all his patients are discretely inarticulate zombies.

It is very important that we should work together, exploit each other's skills ruthlessly so that the patient is always as comfortable as possible, at the same time ensuring that the patient is as much as practicable the person he or she used to be.

We then had some good papers, finding that MST Continus tablets delivered roughly what they said they would deliver: equivalent analgesia for 12 hours, and we had this looked at in different ways. We also learnt as we went along—and to some of us it is a lesson that needs bitterly repeating—that analgesia in inadequate dose is no better than a placebo, and that customer satisfaction (from Mr Paul Jarrett and his day-case herniorraphies) is a reliable way of assessing a regimen of treatment and management that—still to my simple mind—ranks high and is probably the best available at the present time.

Nausea and vomiting remain important problems. We have seen an area of opinion here which says that they tend to dominate the scene most vividly and importantly when analgesia is inadequate or incomplete or the needs for pain relief are smaller.

The patient's control of dosage was, clearly, a concept with which Dr Ian Clarke agreed and enthusiastically involved his patients with, but also raising eyebrows of other doctors. I think that we are going to come to this. I think the patients must, in many western European countries in the next 10 or 20 years, be more closely informed and involved in their own therapeutic regimen. This may not be popular with the doctors, but it is required by the changes of structure in our society. I think we as doctors have to handle the situation or there will be others that will do it worse. I think that we agree with Dr Tim Hunt's presentation about the deleterious effect of additives on the shelf-life of opiate mixtures, thus giving some academic support to what I suspect is widely spread hospice routine: that is, if you are adding things to a simple solution of morphine or diamorphine, and most hospices use nothing else, then that additive is done literally in the medicine glass in the seconds before the patient actually takes the medicine. So that the strawberry and the blackberry flavouring or whatever flavouring of choice is merely added at the time of delivery. This strikes me as something which is perhaps a routine best honoured by its continuance until simple solutions themselves leach away into history.

Dr Henry McQuay's paper supported the idea that morphine disposal might be other than a purely hepatic function, and he implied the possibility of a renal role in low concentration morphine disposal, and certainly produced a very lively discussion which—as lively discussions should do—produced some questions far more important and searching than the answers.

Dr Richard Lamerton reminded us about various basic facts in the home management of terminal cancer cases, and that opiates are the specific treatment for dyspnoea although we are now using—not instead of but as well as—injections of frusemide even in patients very near the end, and we find that this helps the patient in cases of noisy breathing and certainly seems to help the relatives and the nurses.

Dr Geoffrey Hanks reminded us that even hospices find accurate prognoses of survival time not so much difficult as impossible. And, really, having for over 12 years now been Medical Director of the unit where we lose a quarter of our patients within three days of admission, I still am reduced to telling relatives with all the sonorous importance and pomposity that I can command, that I am very experienced in this field and so I know I do not know.

We have had interesting papers on the syringe driver, and epidural morphine, and this allows me to reiterate the importance of different neurolytic techniques being integrated into patient care, so that we can define the bad pain controller as someone who only uses one or two techniques again and again and again . . .

At this stage it is perhaps helpful to bring to your attention Professor Duncan Vere's reminder that truly intractable pain is very rare, that morphine assays we know are still evolving and improving, and that a major task is to change attitudes among the health professionals and—most importantly—among our colleagues. I personally find it rather depressing that the only people who come to the traditional medical meetings are the only people who do not need to attend.

Finally, I would like to thank you, the audience, the 'discussants', the speakers, the chairmen, and our sponsors from Mundipharma in Europe and Napp Laboratories Ltd. in the United Kingdom for what to me has been a delightful and memorable occasion.

I have enjoyed it enormously. At my age and stage, most papers at most meetings can be divided into two categories: the stuff I knew already and the stuff I could not possibly understand. In this case, this proportion was commendably small, I enjoyed myself, I learnt, and I am sure most of us also did.